Bodysnatchers to Lifesavers
Three Centuries of Medicine in Edinburgh

Bodysnatchers to Lifesavers
Three Centuries of Medicine in Edinburgh

TARA WOMERSLEY AND DOROTHY H CRAWFORD

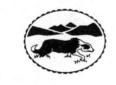

Luath Press Limited

EDINBURGH

www.luath.co.uk

610.9411

First published 2010

ISBN: 978-1-906817-58-9

The paper used in this book is sourced from renewable forestry and is FSC
credited material.

Printed and bound in the UK by MPG Books Ltd, Cornwall

Typeset in 11 point Sabon

Contents

This book is dedicated to the authors' parents,
Ursula and John Womersley and Theo and Margaret Crawford

Acknowledgements

The authors would like to thank the following experts for helpful advice: Mr Mike Barfoot (History of Medicine), Professor Raj Bhopal (Public Health), Professor Andrew Calder (Obstetrics), Dr Maria Dlugolecka-Graham (Polish School of Medicine Memorial Fund); Dr Gordon Findlater (Anatomy), Professor James Garden (Surgery), Professor Ken Murray (Molecular Biology), Professor Kathy Whaler (Geology), Professor Robert Will (Neuroscience) and Professor Lesley Yellowlees (Chemistry). We are also indebted to librarians Ms Laura Bouard (NHS Lothian), Ms Tricia Boyd (University of Edinburgh, Special Collections), Ian Milne (Royal College of Physicians of Edinburgh) and Anne Morrison (Edinburgh City Libraries). In addition the following kindly read and commented on the manuscript: William Alexander, Janet Dalitz, Frances Fowler, Louis Golightley, Ingo Johannessen, Catriona Kelly and Helen Puttick. Mr George Clerk kindly provided photographs.

Foreword

As the latest in a long line of Edinburgh doctors entrusted with stewardship of medical education and research in the city's great international University, it is an honour to introduce this fascinating book. For three centuries medicine in Edinburgh has been no stranger to controversy, but whenever tested, the forces of enlightenment have eventually overcome those of conservatism, whether the issue was the teaching of Anatomy, safe surgery, medical education for women, or human embryonic stem cells. A key factor of 'the Edinburgh Method' has been to base teaching and research firmly in the practice of medicine rather than its theory. This approach has yielded a rich harvest in prevention and cure, and individuals with innovative ideas. In the early 21st century, these values are as strongly held as ever, the only difference being that medical students no longer need instruction in table manners, although this advance needed decades of determined work. So for a story that links Lister with Littlejohn, Simpson with Syme, Darwin with Doyle and Woodruff with Wilmut, read on...

Sir John Savill, BA, MBCHB, PHD, FRCP, FRCPE, FASN, FMedSci, FRSE
Vice-Principal & Head of College of Medicine and Veterinary Medicine, Professor of Experimental Medicine.

Influential Figures in the History of Medicine in Edinburgh

Robert Sibbald	1641–1722
Archibald Pitcairne	1652–1713
Herman Boerhaave	1668–1738
John Monro	1670–1740
Alexander Monro (primus)	1697–1767
James Hutton	1726–1797
Alexander Monro (secundus)	1733–1817
Andrew Duncan	1744–1828
Benjamin Bell	1749–1806
John Barclay	1758–1826
John Bell	1763–1820
Alexander Monro (tertius)	1773–1859
Charles Bell	1774–1842
Richard Bright	1789–1858
William Pulteney Alison	1790–1859
Robert Knox	1791–1862
James Barry	c.1792–1865
Thomas Addison	1793-1860
Robert Liston	1794–1847
Thomas Hodgkin	1798–1866
James Syme	1799–1870
Charles Darwin	1809–1882
John Hughes Bennett	1812–1875
Henry Littlejohn	1826–1914
Hermann Brehmer	1826–1889

Joseph Lister	1827–1912
Isabel Thorne	c.1834–1910
Joseph Bell	1837-1911
Elizabeth Garrett-Anderson	1836–1917
Alex Crum Brown	1838–1932
Sophia Jex-Blake	1840-1912
Robert Koch	1843–1910
Alleyne Nicholson	1844–1899
Edith Pechey	1845–1908
Robert William Philips	1857–1939
Elsie Inglis	1864–1917
Norman Dott	1897–1973
Michael Woodruff	1911–2001
John Crofton	1912–2009
Patrick Forrest	1923–
Kenneth Murray	1931–
Noreen Murray	1935–
Ian Wilmut	1944–

Chronology of Events

1349 The Black Death reaches Edinburgh

1505 The Edinburgh Guild of Barbers and Surgeons established

1582 The University of Edinburgh founded

1603 James VI of Scotland succeeds to the English throne

1657 Edinburgh Town Council creates the Guild of Apothecaries and Surgeons

1670 Robert Sibbald plants a physic garden in Edinburgh

1681 The Royal College of Physicians of Edinburgh granted a Royal charter

1685 Robert Sibbald, James Halket and Archibald Pitcairn appointed joint Professors of the Theory and Practice of Medicine

1707 The Act of Union

1720 Alexander Monro (primus) appointed Professor of Anatomy

1726 The Edinburgh Medical School opens

1729 The 'Little House' hospital opens in Robertson's Close

1741 The Old Infirmary opens in Drummond Place

1755 Joseph Black discovers 'fixed air' – carbon dioxide

1758 Alexander Monro (secondus) succeeds his father as Professor of Anatomy

1765 Building of Edinburgh's New Town commences

1778 The Royal College of Surgeons of Edinburgh granted a Royal charter

1788 James Hutton's *Theory of the Earth* published

1798 Edward Jenner's findings on smallpox vaccination published

1808 Alexander Monro (tertius) succeeds his father as Professor of Anatomy

1811 Charles Bell's *New Idea of the Anatomy of the Brain* published

1813 The Edinburgh Lunatic Asylum opens (later renamed the Royal Edinburgh Hospital)

1812 James Barry graduates in Medicine from the University of Edinburgh

1827 **'Joseph the Miller' murdered in the** West Port by William Burke and William Hare

1830 Charles Bell's *The Nervous System of the Body* published

1831 Major cholera epidemic in Edinburgh

1832 Thomas Hodgkin describes Hodgkin's Disease (Hodgkin's Lymphoma)

1837 Queen Victoria ascends to the throne

1840 James Simpson appointed to the Chair of Midwifery

1842 James Syme carries out the first amputation at the ankle

1845 John Hughes Bennett identifies leukaemia

1847 James Simpson discovers the anaesthetic properties of chloroform

1849 Thomas Addison describes Addison's (Pernicious) Anaemia

1855 Thomas Addison describes Addison's Disease

1859 Charles Darwin's *On the Origin of Species* published

1862 Henry Littlejohn appointed as Edinburgh's first Medical Officer for Health

1865 James Barry dies and is found to be a woman

1865 Littlejohn publishes his report: *On the Sanitary Condition of the City of Edinburgh*

1867 Joseph Lister publishes the results of using carbolic acid as an antiseptic

1869 'The Edinburgh Seven' matriculate at the University of Edinburgh

1869 Lister appointed to the Chair of Clinical Surgery

1870 The first City Fever Hospital opens

1879 The New Royal Infirmary of Edinburgh opens in Lauriston Place

1880 Compulsory notification of infectious diseases introduced in Edinburgh

1885 The second City Fever Hospital opens

1887 Arthur Conan Doyle's *A Study in Scarlet* published

1887 Sophia Jex-Blake opens the Edinburgh School of Medicine for women

1889 Ina and Grace Cadwell and Elsie Inglis set up the Medical College for Women

1894 The University of Edinburgh allows female medical students to graduate

1896 The first female doctors graduate from the University of Edinburgh

1901 King Edward VII ascends to the throne

1903 The City Hospital for Infectious Diseases opens in Colinton Mains

1910 King George V ascends to the throne

1914 **Outbreak of the** First World War

1918 Robert Philip appointed to the first Chair of Tuberculosis

1931 Norman Dott performs the first successful operation on a ruptured brain aneurysm

1939 Outbreak of the Second World War

1939 The Department of Surgical Neurology, known as 'Ward 20', opens at the Royal Infirmary

1941 The Polish School of Medicine established at the University of Edinburgh

1948 The NHS comes into being

1951 John Crofton appointed as Professor of Respiratory Diseases and Tuberculosis

1952 Queen Elizabeth II ascended to the throne

1954 The inauguration of John Crofton's 'Edinburgh Method', which halves TB notifications in the city within four years

1956 The University of Edinburgh sets up a Nursing Teaching Unit

1957 Michael Woodruff appointed as Professor of Surgical Science

1960 Michael Woodruff performs the UK's first successful kidney transplant

1963 The University of Edinburgh establishes the world's first Chair in

General Practice

1971 Patrick Forrest appointed to the Regius Chair of Clinical Surgery

1984 Kenneth Murray's synthetic hepatitis B vaccine becomes available

1986 The first case of BSE – mad cow disease – identified in the UK

1988 The National Breast Cancer Screening programme set up

1990 The National CJD Surveillance Unit set up at the University of Edinburgh

1996 Four deaths from variant CJD reported

1997 Announcement of Dolly the Sheep's birth

2000 Pancreas transplants introduced at the Royal Infirmary of Edinburgh

2002 The Chancellor's Building opens at Little France

2003 The Royal Infirmary of Edinburgh relocates to Little France

2005 The University of Edinburgh's Queen's Medical Research Institute opens at Little France

2008 The Roslin Institute joins with the University of Edinburgh

2010 The Clinical Research Imaging Centre opens

2010 JK Rowling donates £10 million for the Anne Rowling Regenerative Neurology Clinic

Introduction

THE HISTORIES OF Edinburgh and the Medical School of its oldest university have been entwined for centuries in the fight against disease. Today, Edinburgh's medical pioneers find themselves in a new and exciting era as they build on the work of the past and forge ahead with discoveries that will impact on the future. At the University's Little France campus and elsewhere more than 1,000 researchers are pursuing groundbreaking studies with a clear emphasis on translating their findings from the laboratory bench into improved treatments for patients.

Bodysnatchers to Lifesavers looks back to the very roots of medical practice in the city, from the incorporation of the Edinburgh Guild of Barbers and Surgeons in 1505 to the opening of the University's Medical School in 1726 and, shortly after that, the setting up of the city's first teaching hospital – the six-bed 'Little House' in Robertson's Close off the Cowgate.

At the time the Medical School opened, poverty and overcrowding were rife in the city and the lack of sanitation gave free rein to the spread of disease. Death rates were appallingly high, with infants being particularly vulnerable. Scotland's first Medical Officer of Health, Sir Henry Littlejohn, took responsibility for turning the tide of Edinburgh's dreadful public health record. In a long career starting in the mid-19th century, he fought more or less single-handedly for a modern public health system, introducing initiatives such as the compulsory notification of infectious diseases and the provision of free smallpox vaccinations during epidemics.

Public health was not the only aspect of medicine in which Edinburgh established a strong reputation. From the early 18th century the Medical School was renowned for its teaching of Anatomy. This subject was initially dominated by the Monro dynasty, with three generations ruling over the dissecting rooms for more than a hundred years. Their success led to a huge demand for bodies for dissection that was fed by grave-robbers – 'bodysnatchers' – and inspired Burke and Hare to embark on their notorious West Port murder spree.

In the pre-anaesthetic era, surgeons were celebrated for their skill and speed with the knife – for instance, Professor James Syme was reputed to have amputated a leg in 90 seconds. The discovery of the anaesthetic properties of chloroform by James Young Simpson revolutionised surgery by allowing more extensive and invasive techniques, but did little to stem surgical death rates. Operating theatres were often filthy places and now that more time could be spent on operative procedures, patients were at greater risk of post-operative sepsis. It was another surgeon, Joseph Lister, who pioneered the use of the antiseptic carbolic acid, showing that it prevented wounds from becoming infected.

The city's exclusively male medical profession of the 19th century was first infiltrated by one James Barry, who qualified in 1812 and practised as an army doctor for 40 years. Only after her death was it discovered that she was a woman. Shortly after Barry's death 'The Edinburgh Seven', led by the redoubtable Sophia Jex-Blake, mounted a serious assault on the male bastion. Their struggle to follow their calling is a tale of attack, counter-attack, intrigue and underhand manoeuvres.

Famous for teaching the art of astute clinical observation, the Edinburgh Medical School spawned many individuals who, at least in part due to that training, made their names outside medicine. James Hutton deduced that the Earth was not a few thousand but millions of years old, Joseph Black discovered carbon dioxide and Charles Darwin conceived his theory of evolution by natural selection. On the literary front, Arthur Conan Doyle's world-famous detective, Sherlock Holmes, was reputedly modelled on Joseph Bell, the Edinburgh Medical School lecturer whose powers of observation and logical deduction so deeply impressed the author.

These are just a few of the many fascinating episodes recounted in the pages of *Bodysnatchers to Lifesavers* in a story populated with a succession of progressive innovators whose passion, insight and scientific acumen won time and again over blinkered conservatism and petty professional jealousy. While not claiming to be comprehensive, this book reveals the extraordinary human stories behind great developments and charts the impact that advances in medical practice made in Edinburgh has had over the centuries.

CHAPTER I

Medicine in Edinburgh
The Beginning

PERCHED ON ITS VOLCANIC plug high above the city, the castle has dominated the Edinburgh skyline since the 12th century. Edinburgh today is a handsome, thriving capital where most of its 500,000 inhabitants enjoy high standards of hygiene and healthcare, but this has not always been the case. In earlier times the city earned a nickname with a very different resonance: 'Auld Reekie'. For most of its history, privilege and poverty have existed cheek by jowl in this city of contrasts.

In medieval times Edinburgh's main thoroughfare, the Royal Mile, ran along the ridge between the Castle and Holyrood Palace (formerly a monastery), with the Old Town clustered along its length. Narrow wynds ran down to the valleys of the Grassmarket and the Cowgate to the west and south respectively, and to the north to the Nor Loch, which served as the city's water supply and sewage dump and, in the 16th century, as a convenient spot for 'douking' suspected witches. In the warren of narrow, dank wynds, the rich lived alongside the poor, inhabiting tenements that rose as high as 14 storeys, often with whole families accommodated in each tiny room. Class distinction in medieval Edinburgh was vertical rather than horizontal, with the better-off in the brighter, airier upper storeys and the poorest packed into the darkest, dampest, most polluted corners, often underground. Water had to be carried from street pumps and all sewage and refuse was simply thrown into the wynds and left to slither down the steep passageways. Sewage disposal took place daily on the dot of 10pm. When the bell of St Giles

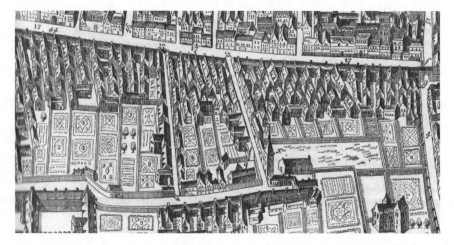

The Cowgate area in 1646, showing 'Robertson's Wynd' (no.54) where the six-bed 'Little House', the first teaching hospital in Edinburgh, opened in 1729.

chimed, doors and windows flew open and, to the call of 'Gardez loo!', all those in the street ran for cover as rubbish was thrown down from above.

In comparison to its southerly neighbour, medieval Scotland was a poor country and in the 16th and 17th centuries the streets of Edinburgh saw riots caused by food shortages, poor pay and housing conditions, unemployment and destitution. The capital was also torn by religious and political strife between Jacobites and Hanoverians, pro- and anti-Unionists, and Catholics and Protestants. As its population grew – from 25,000 in 1600 to 50,000 in 1750 – nothing was done to relieve the overcrowding and living conditions deteriorated for the less well-off. With no poor relief to stave off food shortages and no basic hygiene to prevent epidemics, it is no wonder that Auld Reekie was a very unhealthy place to live.

When James VI of Scotland succeeded to the English throne (as James I) in 1603, many courtiers and noblemen followed him south, leaving the capital bereft. By the time of the Act of Union in 1707, an air of depression and lethargy had settled over Edinburgh. National commerce had stagnated, causing a serious downturn in international trade. After the failed 1745 rebellion the Union was broadly accepted as irreversible, even by many who had supported the Jacobite cause, and its advantages were becoming evident, as it brought much-needed wealth to Scotland through imperial trade with the West and East Indies and North America. Some of the Scottish nobility returned and a wealthy merchant class began to dominate the scene. Beginning around 1730, the cultural renaissance known as the Scottish Enlightenment placed Edinburgh at the centre of intellectual life in Europe. An extraordinary number of eminent thinkers congregated in the city, including the philosopher David Hume, the novelist Sir Walter Scott and the poet Robert Burns. An ambitious town-planning project saw the building of the New Town commence in 1765. As part of this development the highly polluted Nor Loch was drained, to reveal the bodies of several suspected witches who were proved innocent posthumously by the fact that they had drowned (the belief was that real witches would float). The construction of bridges spanning the valleys to the north and south allowed further expansion of the city and many of the better-off moved to the New Town. The neoclassical style of its streets, terraces and squares, and the intellectual vibrancy of the period earned Edinburgh the name of 'the Athens of the North'.

The lot of the poor in the Old Town did not improve, as any space created by the exodus of the well-heeled was soon filled by immigrants, particularly the destitute from Ireland, who came seeking employment. The enormous movement from countryside to city during the Industrial Revolution meant that crowding only got worse and poverty, famine and disease all took their toll. Smallpox, cholera, tuberculosis (TB) and other infections were frequent visitors. With no idea how to control or treat them and no organised medical services, citizens succumbed to these diseases right up until the early 20th century.

The University of Edinburgh

Established in 1582, the University of Edinburgh differed from its rivals, Oxford, Cambridge, Aberdeen and St Andrews in that it was set up by the Town Council and not the Church. Referred to as the 'Toun's College', this lack of religious affiliation had many advantages in a time of religious conflict but in the political upheavals that followed the College was left severely underfunded. There was no organised building programme until the magnificent buildings of Old College were designed by Robert Adam in the late 18th century and completed by William Playfair in the early 19th century.

In the early days University teachers, known as 'regents', were paid so little that many quickly found more lucrative employment elsewhere. A regent's annual stipend of 40 merks (around £27) plus board and student fees (£2 per course for townsfolk, £3 for outsiders, paid directly to the teacher) contrasted poorly with that of a parish minister, making the Church an attractive alternative.[1] Students, who began their studies at the age of 13 or 14, were taught all subjects throughout their four years at University by the same regent. Since the regent's income depended on the number of students taught, staff-to-student ratios were high. This led to overcrowded lectures for the most popular teachers – not a great recipe for student satisfaction. Wealthy citizens preferred to send their sons abroad to study, principally to Padua in the 16th century and to Utrecht or Leiden in the 17th. In Leiden a revolution in teaching methods was under way, spearheaded by the charismatic Herman Boerhaave, who had read Philosophy and later Medicine there, and

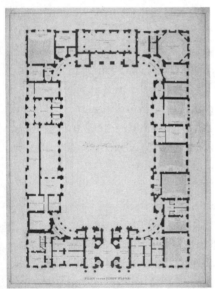

Plans of Old College showing the Anatomy lecture theatre in the North West corner (from *The Student* 1885–1903).

was appointed Professor of Botany and Medicine in 1709. In 1714 he became Rector of Leiden University and also Professor of Practical Medicine and revolutionised teaching practices by abolishing regents and introducing specialist teaching that for the first time allowed professors to stick entirely to their own subjects, although their stipend still depended on the number of students they attracted. Boerhaave, whose teaching methods brought him fame throughout Europe in his own lifetime, continued to practise medicine as well as teach it. In 1724 he described the case of Baron Jan von Wassenaer, a Dutch admiral who died of a ruptured oesophagus caused by severe vomiting after indulging in a gluttonous feast – an unpleasant end to an enjoyable meal. The condition, which was universally fatal at the time, is still known as 'Boerhaave's Syndrome'.[2]

Boerhaave's innovations in teaching methods swept Europe. The University of Edinburgh abandoned the regenting system in 1708, around the same time as plans for a new Medical School reached fruition. Its reputation as an international centre of learning grew as the century progressed and students came from far and wide, particularly to attend courses at the Medical School which was by then the dominant Faculty. 'No place in the world can pretend to compete with Edinburgh', American President Thomas Jefferson commented in 1789.[3]

The University, a popular choice for children of the Scottish diaspora, also became a haven for the politically marginalised; it welcomed those affected by the French Revolution and the Napoleonic Wars, English nonconformists banned from the ecclesiastical universities of Oxford and Cambridge, and Irish Presbyterians excluded from Dublin.

The Edinburgh Medical School

The practice of medicine in medieval Edinburgh was at best primitive and at worst positively dangerous, with all classes dependant on traditional herbal remedies. By the 18th century quackery abounded and the rich often fell prey to impostors purveying expensive potions that had no curative value. One such charlatan was James Graham, a charismatic individual who studied Medicine at the University but by all accounts dropped out before qualifying. Graham practised medicine illegally in England before making a visit to America from which he returned extolling the healing powers of electricity and magnetism. His claim that 'electricity invigorates the whole body and remedies all physical defects' brought rich patrons flocking to his lavishly appointed 'Temple of Health' in London's Pall Mall. There, attended by 'goddesses of health' (one of whom was Emma Hart, the future Lady Hamilton and mistress of Horatio Nelson), they wallowed in electrically charged baths or slept in 'celestial beds' surrounded by powerful magnets (offered as a cure for infertile couples).

Interest in Graham's novel 'cures' eventually waned in London. With his debts rising, in 1783 he returned to Edinburgh, where one of his customers was the 14-year-old Walter Scott, who had suffered from polio and was referred to Graham by his maternal grandfather, a doctor. Over the years Graham became increasingly eccentric and was eventually committed as insane.[4] To be charitable, the purported remedies offered by this flamboyant character were probably no less effective than some other unlikely 'cures' which were nonetheless apparently mainstream, such as this one for colic:

> The hoofs of living creatures are good, being drunk; or dry ox-dung in broth, or the juice pressed from ox-dung drunk is better. The heart of a lark bound to the thigh is excellent against colic; and some have eaten it raw with good success.[5]

From early times care of the sick and destitute in Scotland, as in other European countries, was provided by monks who ran hospitals for the needy. In Scotland the largest of these was at Soutra Hill, about 18 miles south-east of Edinburgh, where a church, Augustinian friary and hospital complex known as the 'House of the Holy Trinity' was granted a royal charter by Malcolm IV in 1164. Seeds from medicinal herbs such as henbane, hemlock and even the non-British opium poppy have been excavated at the site, where many early surgical instruments have also been found. The hospital's proximity to the Via Regia, the main north–south road, meant that the hospital, which remained open until the 17th century, tended not only the local poor and sick, but also travellers including pilgrims and soldiers.

Following a papal edict in 1215 forbidding monks to have direct contact with blood, the holy practitioners enlisted barbers to assist in procedures such as bone-setting, tooth-drawing and stone-cutting, as well as the common practice of bleeding out evil humours. This unlikely alliance was the origin of the Edinburgh Guild of Barbers and Surgeons, which was approved by the Town Council in 1505 in an attempt to oust quacks. From then on, would-be practitioners had to learn their skills by apprenticeship to a master and gain a licence.

In contrast to barber-surgeons, physicians can trace their history to apothecaries and pharmacists whose trade of concocting and dispensing drugs and potions was often handed down through the generations along with folklore and herbal remedies. This branch of the profession had no guild until 1657 when the Town Council created a single Guild of Apothecaries and Surgeons. The alliance was fragile and uneasy. Competition was fierce and jealousy abounded. The physician was recognised as a gentleman, the surgeon more as a tradesman.[6]

A separate College of Physicians was granted a royal charter in 1681 and a charter for the College of Surgeons followed in 1778. The Royal Colleges, like the joint Guild of Apothecaries and Surgeons before them, trained by apprenticeship and granted a licence to practise after examination.

At the start of the 18th century a group of 'Leiden men', inspired by Boerhaave, were keen to set up a medical school in Edinburgh using his teaching methods. A leading advocate of this system was Robert Sibbald, a physician-apothecary from Fife who planted a physic garden in Edinburgh in 1670 to encourage the study of Botany and Materia Medica (Pharmacy). Sibbald recounts in his autobiography:

So I had from my settlement here in Edinburgh a designe to informe myself of the natural history thus resolved to make it part of my study to know those animals, vegetables, mineralls, metals and substances cast up by the sea, were found in this country, that might be of use in medicine, or other artes usefull to human lyfe.[7]

In 1685 Edinburgh Town Council appointed Sibbald and two of his colleagues, James Halket and Archibald Pitcairne (who had been Professor of Medicine in Leiden prior to Boerhaave) as professors of the Theory and Practice of Medicine. Twenty years later, in 1705, a Chair of Anatomy was established. Extraordinary as it may seem, none of these professorships involved any teaching – it was not until professors of Botany, Chemistry, Materia Medica and Midwifery were appointed and the Medical School proper opened in 1726, that comprehensive training leading to a degree in medicine was inaugurated. The University teachers were in competition with private teaching establishments, so-called 'extra-mural' schools, most of which were clustered around the University in Surgeons' Square, and taught students heading for exams at the Colleges of Physicians and Surgeons or for the University degree.

The three-year Doctor of Medicine (MD) degree course included Anatomy, Surgery, Chemistry, Botany, Materia Medica, and the Theory and Practice of Medicine. Teaching in clinical medicine was conducted in the six-bedded Infirmary, 'the Little House', which opened in Robertson's Close off the Cowgate in 1729 in premises rented from the Town Council. Run by public subscription, it was replaced within 20 years by 'the Old Infirmary' in Drummond Street. This building, designed by William Adam, could accommodate more than 200 patients. This allowed the emphasis on practical, hospital-based teaching which became Edinburgh's hallmark and gained the Medical School an excellent reputation for clinical tuition.

To gain the MD degree students had to submit a thesis on a medical topic. At the end of the course they were obliged to present themselves, suitably attired in a black silk waistcoat, for a final oral examination conducted by at least two professors, covering all medical disciplines and including a detailed discussion of two cases. Until 1833 the thesis was written, and the examination conducted, entirely in Latin. This rigorous procedure was generally regarded as necessary for physicians, but budding surgeons often preferred to take the more practical College of Surgeons' licentiate diploma.

These extra-mural schools, including the Colleges of Physicians and Surgeons, provided intense competition for the University teachers. The colleges continued to offer medical qualifications until 1948, but it was in the 18th century that the rivalry between the University's medical professors and the extra-mural teachers was strongest, with students attending the cheaper extra-mural classes according to their needs, ambitions, finances and whim. In the first 20 years of the Medical School's existence only 36 students graduated with MD degrees,[8] and during the whole 18th century larger numbers qualified from the extra-mural schools than the University MD course.[9]

The 1745 Jacobite rebellion and almost continuous warfare on the Continent meant that the majority of beds in the infirmary were filled with military casualties and, not surprisingly, many Edinburgh graduates chose to join the army or the navy. Indeed at one time the vast majority of army doctors were Scottish and most of these were Edinburgh trained.[10] Whether the military were grateful for this we do not know, but they did insist on potential recruits spending time at the General Hospital, Fort Pitt, at Chatham, living in the mess at their own expense – not least, to learn table manners. One recruit later wrote:

The medical service was then principally recruited from Scotch and Irish schools, some of them very rough specimens, who were entirely innocent at first of the ordinary uses of a silver fork or finger-basin at dinner, and whose period of probation at a military mess-table was not the least useful part of their education; but under this rather uncultivated exterior there were not a few instances of those who, in their subsequent career, gave testimony that they possessed a high sense of duty, and a lofty estimate of the purpose of life.[11]

At the outset the University of Edinburgh made no attempt to provide college accommodation for students as at Oxford and Cambridge. This was not to everyone's liking, as Captain Edward Topham, who stayed in Edinburgh for several months in 1774–75, remarked in his *Letters from Edinburgh*:

... [the students] are under no restraint from the College but have lodgings in the City. In general they are very extravagant, especially those from Ireland, who too often forsake the calm retired paths of learning and science to revel in public scenes of dissipation and debauchery. But the students who are natives of this country present a different picture. The miserable holes which some of them inhabit, their abstemiousness and parsimony, their constant attendance to study, their indefatigable industry, even border on romance.[12]

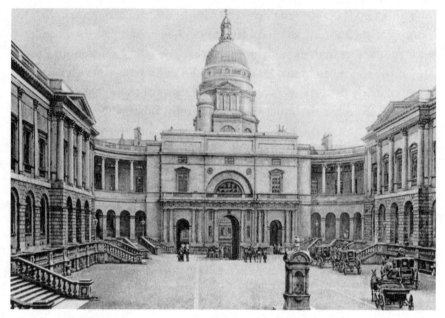

The quadrangle of Old College (picture from *The Student* 1885–1903).

Although surgical apprentices generally lived with their masters and students sometimes lodged with their professor's family, in general students' experience of Edinburgh varied according to their means and background. The wealthiest enjoyed all the cultural and social advantages of the city, while poor students often suffered in cold, damp, unhealthy lodgings in the wynds around the University. The contrast was stark, as Professor Andrew Duncan junior remarked in the early 1800s:

> I have known instances of students getting through the winter on less than £10 [equivalent to around £500 today]; I have known other medical students spend almost £500 or £600.[13]

Most medical students worked hard, being occupied from 8am to 7pm with lectures, anatomy demonstrations and examining patients in the infirmary. The journal of one student who attended classes between 1771 and 1772 reveals a programme of rigorous study. He rose at 7, read till 8, then attended a Chemistry lecture before breakfasting at 9. He wrote up his notes from 10 till noon, visited the wards from noon till 1 and attended the anatomy department from 1–3. He then dined in his lodging before a lecture on midwifery from 4–5, writing his notes from 5–6, attending an anatomical demonstration from 6–7 and taking supper at 9. He then studied in his lodgings before going to bed at midnight.[14]

Anatomy and the Monros

The Monro family ruled the anatomy dissecting rooms of Edinburgh for 128 years, from 1720 to 1848, with father, son and grandson – Monro primus, secundus and tertius – holding the Chair of Anatomy in straight succession.

The story of the Monro dynasty begins with Monro primus's father, John Monro from Stirling, who studied Medicine under Pitcairne in Leiden and practised as a surgeon in William of Orange's army before retiring his commission and becoming a surgeon-apothecary in Edinburgh. He was influential, serving as Treasurer and Deacon of the Incorporation of Surgeons from 1712 to 1713. He was one of those who dreamt of establishing a medical school in Edinburgh fashioned after the Leiden model and he tailored his son Alexander's education so that he could take a prominent role in it. Alexander Monro studied Anatomy, Chemistry and Botany while apprenticed to his father in Edinburgh before travelling to London in 1717 where he had his first opportunity to dissect human bodies. He then studied in Paris for a short while before proceeding to Leiden to gain his MD under Boerhaave's tuition, returning to Edinburgh in 1719. Shortly after his election to the College of Surgeons, John McGill and Adam Drummond, the joint professors of Anatomy, resigned in his favour, citing poor health and pressure of other commitments, but doubtless pushed by Monro senior.

Monro primus assumed the title of Professor of Anatomy in 1720 at the tender age of 22. Then father and son, with the help of their influential friend, George Drummond, Lord Provost of Edinburgh, set about founding the Infirmary in Robertson's Close which was essential for Leiden-style clinical teaching, and where Monro primus regularly taught his students. By all accounts he was a charismatic and inspiring teacher, attracting crowds to his lectures – fortunate, since the student lecture fees augmented his salary of just £15 a year. Soon his lectures and demonstrations, delivered in the Anatomy Theatre in Old Surgeon's Hall, were attracting more than 300 students and had to be repeated at a second sitting. Attendees included students from the University and the extra-mural schools, some of whom enrolled for two or three consecutive years, and enthusiasts who had no intention of studying medicine at all. Clearly a man of ability and energy, Monro primus had a thriving private practice in the town to augment his income and was also a prolific writer, with a famous treatise entitled *The Anatomy of Human Bones* and the six-volume *Medical Essays and Observations* to his name.

Although formally it was the role of the Town Council to appoint professors at the University, at this time holders – including Monro primus – took on the task of finding a successor, often handing on the baton to a family member. Monro primus had earmarked his second son, also called Alexander, for the professorship and educated him accordingly. Monro secundus studied Medicine in Edinburgh, assisting in some of his father's Anatomy teaching while still a student. He then went to London, where he worked at St George's Hospital with the famous anatomist and obstetrician William Hunter, and later studied in Berlin and Leiden.

He returned home to take the Chair of Anatomy and Surgery in 1758 after his father resigned because of ill health. Monro secundus held the Chair for the next 40 years and was without a doubt the most influential anatomist of his time. Apparently even more able than his father, he was a wonderful teacher, an excellent administrator and a gifted researcher, who also found time for private practice. His research on the lymphatic system led him to believe (mistakenly) that it was a closed, absorbent system separate from the blood, but publication of his thesis, *De venis lymphaticis valvosis,* in Berlin in 1757 enraged his former mentor, Hunter, who accused him of plagiarism. Monro secundus insisted that the reverse was true.

In fact, the existence of an earlier publication on the subject indicates that neither produced the original idea. Monro's place in medical history was secured by his identification of tiny holes which allow fluid to flow

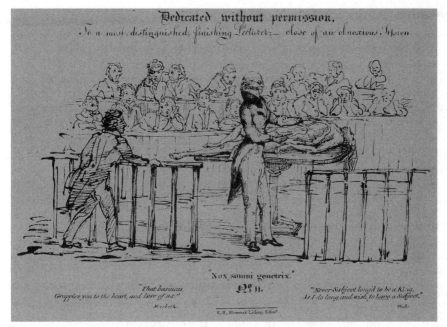

Cartoon of surgeon and anatomist Robert Knox conducting an autopsy.

from one side of the brain to the other between the lateral ventricles, the so-called 'Foramen of Monro'.[15]

In the tradition of the times, Monro secundus was succeeded by his eldest son, also Alexander. Monro tertius, who held the Chair from 1808 until 1848, is said to have been an indifferent lecturer who often read verbatim from his grandfather's notes.[16] The students responded in the customary manner, making their disapproval known by jeering and hurling peas![17] To be fair, the achievements of his forebears set the bar very high and there was now severe competition from the extra-mural schools where two brilliant Anatomy lecturers, Robert Knox and John Barclay, vastly outshone him.

One of his students, the young Charles Darwin, wrote dismissively that he 'made his lectures on human anatomy as dull as he was himself', adding that the subject 'disgusted' him. Darwin also commented on Monro turning up to lectures still covered in blood from a dissection: 'I dislike him & his lectures so much that I cannot speak with decency about them. He is so dirty in person & actions.'[18] It would seem that

Monro tertius is amongst those who can be credited with putting Darwin off his medical studies – allowing his interests to flow instead towards natural history, to the benefit of us all.

Fame and Infamy

Today the study of anatomy remains an essential part of basic medical training, but in the 18th century it was also the subject of intense research. The use of human bodies for research and teaching was relatively new – previous generations of medical practitioners made do with the bodies of animals. Human dissection was controversial. Influenced by religious doctrine, many found it abhorrent. Edinburgh Town Council appreciated the need for human anatomical dissection in medical training, particularly for would-be surgeons, and as early as 1505 granted the Incorporation of Barbers and Surgeons the body of one executed criminal a year on which to teach human anatomy and use for examining apprentices on completion of their training. During this examination, which took place over a four to five day period, the candidate had to demonstrate his surgical skills by undertaking an operation on the dead body. But one body a year was far from adequate. In the late 17th century the Town Council agreed to provide additional bodies – of prisoners who had died or been executed – once the College of Surgeons had built a lecture theatre where they could be dissected before a large audience. Old Surgeon's Hall (now demolished), was completed in 1697 and the first annual public dissection, of a hanged criminal, took place there in 1702. This event took eight days to complete with each system being dissected by a different surgeon over the first seven days, and an epilogue from Pitcairne, Professor of Medicine, on the last.[19] Anatomists and surgeons could now apply to the Town Council for bodies for the purposes of teaching students and apprentices, and it was in Old Surgeon's Hall that Monro primus taught to an ever-increasing and enthusiastic audience.

There is no doubt that the very popularity of Anatomy at the time was instrumental in encouraging resurrectionism – the practice of grave-robbing. As the student audience grew, the demand for bodies outstripped supply and a black market trade in corpses blossomed, fed by this grisly but lucrative occupation. Bodysnatchers operated under cover of darkness, digging up recently buried coffins and transporting the cadaver to an Anatomy theatre in an innocuous-looking sack. To counter this threat, wealthy relatives set their loved ones in iron cases, surrounded graves with iron railings and mounted guards, but still the practice continued. In the words of Sir Robert Christison, Professor of Medicine in Edinburgh in the 1820s:

> The time chosen in the dark winter nights was from 6–8 o'clock, at which late hour the churchyard watch was set, and the city police also commenced their night rounds. A hole was dug down to the coffin only where the head lay – a canvas sheet being stretched around to receive the earth, and to prevent any of its spoiling the smooth uniformity of the grass. The digging was done with short, flat, dagger-shaped implements of wood, to avoid the clicking noise of iron striking stones. On reaching the coffin two broad iron hooks under the lid, pulled up forcibly with a rope, broke off a sufficient portion of the lid to allow the body to be dragged out, and sacking was heaped over the whole to deaden the sound of the creaking wood. The whole process could be completed in an hour, even though the grave might be 6ft deep, because the soil was loose, and the digging was done impetuously by frequent relays of active men.[20]

Rumours that grave-robbing was supplying the city's anatomy theatres spread and in 1725 riots broke out. An angry mob threatened to destroy Old Surgeon's Hall while Monro primus was lecturing to his students, an episode that prompted him to retreat to the safer surroundings of the University buildings. From then on he taught in the University and petitioned the Town Council to provide an Anatomy theatre within the University's gates. Once constructed, this served well until Monro secundus's popularity meant that his class outgrew it and in 1764 he asked for a 200-seat lecture theatre. His request was eventually granted, but only after he had offered £300 towards its cost, to be repaid in instalments by the Town Council. His theatre was eventually demolished in 1793 to make way for the Old College buildings, where all medical teaching took place until the 1870s. The Anatomy Department in the north-west corner of Old College was the first part of the whole building to be completed and occupied. It contained an octagonal, two-storey lecture theatre. A subterranean passageway that still runs under Chambers Street (formerly North College Street) was originally used for transporting bodies from the receiving room near the hospital to the department.[21]

Extra-mural Competition

In 1800, after gaining an MD from Edinburgh, John Barclay set up a School of Anatomy, complete with teaching and dissecting rooms, at 10 Surgeon's Square. Under the inspiring tutelage of Monro secundus he developed a special interest in Comparative Anatomy. By all accounts he was an excellent teacher. After his course of lectures was formally recognised by the College of Surgeons in 1804 it became increasingly popular; by the time he retired from ill health in 1825, it was attended by more than 300 students a year. His successor, Robert Knox, was one of his former students.

The demand for bodies so that students attending Barclay's school could gain experience of dissecting far outstripped local supply. Extra bodies were acquired when and where they became available, most coming from Ireland via Liverpool. Some also came from St Thomas's Hospital in London, where the porter responsible for receiving them was prepared, for a price, to reroute them to Edinburgh.[22]

Knox became heavily implicated in these dubious practices. He had graduated from Edinburgh in 1814, entered the Army Medical Department and spent some time in Brussels and South Africa before studying Anatomy in Paris, a city where unclaimed corpses were freely available for dissection and grave-robbing was unknown. Knox returned to Edinburgh in 1822, became Barclay's partner in the Anatomy School in 1825 and that same year took over from his mentor, whose teaching style he emulated – with the addition of a sharp wit which was often used at the expense of his medical colleagues, gaining him some influential enemies. Knox's lectures became so renowned both for their instructive

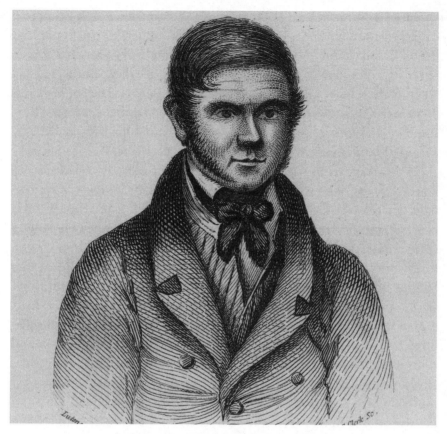

Portrait of William Burke by T Clerk and Lutenor.

and entertainment value that by the late 1820s he was teaching a class of more than 500. From 1826 dissection was made a compulsory part of the medical curriculum and although some of those signed up for his lectures were artists and scholars with no intention of acquiring an MD, and therefore no need to dissect, Knox still needed around 90 cadavers a year. In 1827 he found a new supply line when two local characters by the names of William Burke and William Hare came to him claiming to have bought the bodies they were offering from relatives of the deceased. But according to the Anatomy School doorkeeper, David Patterson, in his evidence at Burke's trial, when removed from the tea chest in which they were delivered the bodies showed unmistakable signs of suffocation or strangulation.[23]

Burke and Hare had come to Scotland from Ireland in search of employment. Both had worked as labourers on the construction of the Union Canal. Later Hare and his common-law wife, Margaret Laird, ran a boarding house in Edinburgh's West Port, where Burke and his common-law wife, Helen MacDougal, often lodged. During a period of 11 months between 1827 and 1828, assisted by their partners, they committed at least 15 murders and sold the bodies for between £7 and £15 to Knox's Anatomy School.

The enterprise began with a tempting opportunity when one of Hare's tenants died while owing him the sum of £4. Perhaps it seemed only fair to steal the body from its coffin and sell it to Knox for the princely sum of £7. Then, with the promise of easy money, the killing spree known as the West Port murders began.

The first victim was 'Joseph the Miller', another tenant at the lodging house, who was sick enough to ply with alcohol and suffocate. Burke and Hare next resorted to preying upon vulnerable individuals picked up off the street. The victims were lured to the lodging house, often by Laird and MacDougal; Burke and Hare then killed them and transported the cadavers to the School of Anatomy. The killers came close to exposure on a couple of occasions: medical students recognised the body of a prostitute, Mary Patterson, and that of 'Daft Jamie', a lad who was well known in the area. Discovery eventually came when the body of Mary Docherty – lured to the boarding house by Burke, who claimed to be her relative – was discovered under a bed by lodgers James and Ann Gray. Although the body had been removed by the time the police arrived, it was eventually found at Knox's Anatomy School and identified by the Grays.

Despite the large number of murders committed, most of the bodies had been dissected and the remains disposed of, so firm evidence was scant. It was not until Hare turned king's evidence, so gaining immunity from prosecution, that there was enough evidence for Burke and MacDougal to go to trial. The case against MacDougal was found 'not proven' and she was released. Burke was condemned to death and was hanged before a jeering crowd in the Lawnmarket in January 1829. After his release Hare disappeared without trace. More remains of both

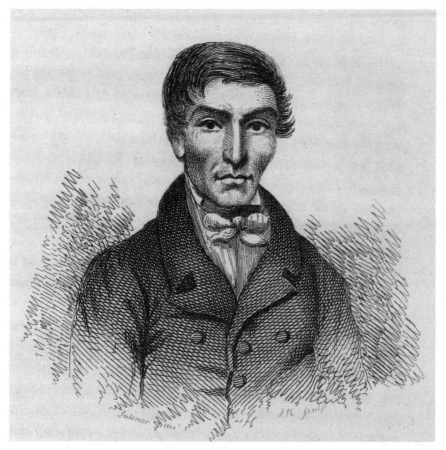

Portrait of William Hare by JR and Lutenor.

Burke and Hare than their reputations alone – the Anatomy Museum has a life mask of Hare and the death mask and skeleton of Burke, and a notebook cover made of Burke's skin is held at the Royal College of Surgeons of Edinburgh. Robert Knox was not called to give evidence at the trial, although afterwards he was questioned by a Committee of Distinguished Citizens who, after a six week investigation, concluded:

> ... by this laxity of the regulations under which bodies were received into his rooms, [Knox] unintentionally gave a degree of familiarity to the disposal of the victims of their crimes, which under better regulations would not have existed.[24]

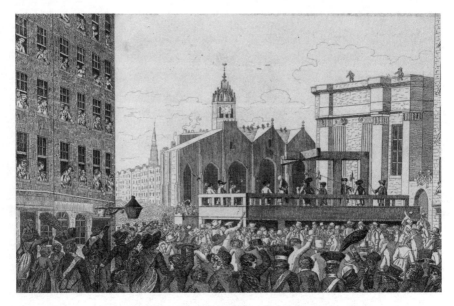

Execution of the notorious William Burke.

Following these events, Knox continued to lecture to a dwindling cohort of students but he had lost all support from his medical colleagues, many of whom had been ridiculed in his lectures, and was extremely unpopular in the town at large. He gave up teaching in the Anatomy School in 1833 and eventually moved to London, where he took up the post of Consulting Physician at the Brompton Hospital and died in relative poverty at the age of 71.

The West Port murders attracted wide press interest and aroused considerable revulsion; clearly something had to be done to prevent a repeat of such a barbaric episode of medical history. There is no doubt that the public disquiet engendered by the murders acted as the impetus for the UK government to draw up the Anatomy Act which became law in 1832. This at last provided for a tightly regulated, legal supply of cadavers for medical dissection and remained in place until superseded by the Anatomy Act of 1984 which, in Scotland, has now been amended by the Human Tissue Act of 2006.

From his vantage point in Old College, Monro tertius watched the events of 1827–28 unfold. He documented them in a scrapbook, now held in the University of Edinburgh library, which contains a poem written at the time of the trial by 'Wag Phil', which mentions Knox as K.........; although humorous, this 'Timely Hint' underscores the immense public concern over this tragic affair.

A Timely Hint to Anatomical Practitioners and their
Associates – the Resurrectionists.[25]

A New Song
Tune, Macpherson's Farewell

What is our land at last come to
Our ancestors would weep,
And say, with many, were they here,
'Look well before ye leap'.

Ye prowling Resurrectionists
Of every clime and shore,
Remember Burke, that smoth'ring wretch,
For he is now no more.

This monster, with his meagre chief,
In action mean and low,
Resolv'd to rid the land of all
That wandered to and fro.

Two buxom females, with those brutes,
In this work had their share
One party coax'd them to the den,
The other slew them there.

They with the greatest kindness wiled
Daft Jamie off the street,
Whose playful manner did delight
All that he chanced to meet.

With Judas smiles they did betray
The aged Dougherty
Who wander'd long from door to door
In search of charity.

MacDougal, Patterson, and more,
Were by those fiends beguil'd,
Nor did they shudder to destroy
The helpless smiling child.

Men, women, children old and young,
The sickly and the hale,
Were murder'd, pack'd up and sent off
To K.........'s human sale.

That man of skill, with subjects warm,
Was frequently supplied
Nor did he question when or how
The person brought had died!

If he wants subjects let him try
From France to get them o'er
For he can get them, when he will,
Sent at Six pounds the score.

Or let him try some legal means
His subjects to obtain,
Nor even more in word or deed
Wink at such tricks again.

One of the tribe has met his fate
On gibbet high and strong,
And if such pranks are play'd again,
The rest will swing o'er long.

CHAPTER 2

Surgery, Anaesthesia and Antisepsis

DURING THE 18TH and early 19th centuries, Anatomy was considered of prime importance, overshadowing Surgery as a specialty in its own right. Historically surgeons had to make house calls through the servant's entrance of patients' homes, while the respected physicians would be welcomed at the front door, a practice that reflected the comparatively humble position of surgeons in society. In Edinburgh such a distinction between surgery and anatomy appears to have been maintained by the Monro dynasty. Although Monro primus held the Chair of Anatomy, Monros secundus and tertius both held the combined Chairs of Anatomy and Surgery but neither practised much surgery.

Surgery in Edinburgh entered a new era when, in 1802, the first Chair of Clinical Surgery was established, founded by King George III. Four years later a Chair of Military Surgery was inaugurated. The first of its kind in Britain, it was seen as a way to prepare medical students and practitioners for the front line. This Chair was to remain in existence for less than 50 years with just two holders; ironically it was abolished when the Crimean War was at its height. The establishment of a Chair of Systematic Surgery in 1831 was perhaps a contributory factor in the demise of Military Surgery as a discipline. There was also now much more of a focus on the practice of surgery than simply the theory behind it.

In the 1800s Edinburgh surgeons had begun to make names for themselves. Benjamin Bell, one such surgeon, is regarded by many as the 'father of the Edinburgh surgical school'. While the Monros were physicians without surgical training, Bell did much to establish Edinburgh's reputation as a centre for surgical teaching. Born into a landowning family from Dumfriesshire, he was apprenticed to a local surgeon after leaving school. The experience was to serve him in good stead when in 1766 he enrolled at the Edinburgh Medical School, then working as a surgical dresser and surgeon's clerk at the Royal Infirmary. After furthering his studies in London and Paris, he returned to Edinburgh and at the tender age of 24 was appointed as surgeon to the Royal Infirmary. His surgical career was almost curtailed after a horse-riding accident from which he spent almost two years recovering. He was said to have contemplated abandoning surgery altogether, having leased a farm at Liberton, outside Edinburgh, with the idea that this might become his livelihood.[1]

Fortunately Bell returned to surgery, for he was to make a significant impact on surgical techniques. He realised that problems relating to how wounds healed after amputations often resulted because of insufficient skin and muscle flaps. His maxim 'save skin' helped the healing process.[2] Before the era of anaesthetics, Bell stressed the importance of reducing the pain endured by patients during surgery. He turned to homeopathy as well as advocating the use of opium as an analgesic. His standing was such that a contemporary wrote, 'nobody could die contented without having consulted Benjamin Bell.'[3] His vision of writing a guide to surgical management and technique was realised in his celebrated work *A System of Surgery*, published in six volumes between 1783 and 1788. The work was the first comprehensive textbook of surgery in English. Other groundbreaking works by Bell, a prolific author, include *A Treatise on Gonorrhoea Virukenta and Lues Venera* (1793), in which he observed that the causes and clinical features of gonorrhoea and syphilis were different, contradicting the belief that there was only a single venereal disease, and *A Treatise on the Hydrocele, or Sarcocele, or Cancer and Other Diseases of the Testes* (1801). His legacy lived on not only in his writings but also with a family dynasty of surgeons. His two sons George and Joseph Bell became surgeons, as did their sons, who were both called Benjamin. His great-grandson, Joseph, also a surgeon, was Sir Arthur Conan Doyle's inspiration for Sherlock Holmes.

Other eminent Edinburgh surgeons to follow Bell were James Syme and his mentor and subsequent adversary, Robert Liston, whose practices also began in the pre-anaesthesia era when patients, with only alcohol to dull the terrible pain inflicted by the surgeon's knife, often had to be physically restrained. Surgical skill and speed were of the essence. The microbial cause of post-operative sepsis was unknown (the germ theory only became widely accepted in the 19th century), but surgeons were acutely aware of the prevalence of post-operative deaths and so it is not surprising that invasive surgery was generally restricted to life-saving procedures.

Syme, who in his prime was able to amputate a leg in 90 seconds,[4] grew up in a grand house in the New Town and enrolled at the University in 1815 at the age of 16, already certain that he wanted to be a doctor. Like many of his contemporaries he began by studying Latin, essential for Medicine. His first year of medical studies included Chemistry. While many today may not have heard of Syme, his chemical prowess could easily have made him a household name. In 1818 he managed to make a silk coat rain-resistant by using naphtha as a solvent for rubber, which could then waterproof the cloth. Five years later Charles Mackintosh from Glasgow patented a similar process, earning himself a fortune. Syme never received a penny and raincoats became known as mackintoshes rather than symes.

As a student Syme was impressed by the lectures of Robert Liston, a distant cousin, who was renowned for his surgical skill and speed. However, Liston's speed did not always work for the best. Following one amputation which lasted less than two and a half minutes, not only did the patient die from gangrene but so did one of Liston's assistants, after the surgeon accidentally severed his fingers. A third man, who was simply observing, 'expired from hysteria, thinking Liston had punctured his internal organs when only his coat had been cut.'[5]

Liston had an abrasive manner that failed to endear him to his colleagues and his reputation as a difficult character was not helped when he became the subject of public controversy because of his disapproval

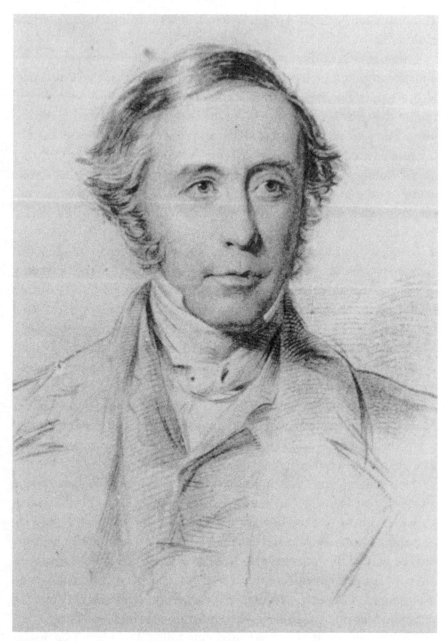

James Syme.

of the way the Royal Infirmary of Edinburgh was run. Syme became his assistant and demonstrator in 1818 and eventually took charge of his anatomy class in 1823, but the pair quarrelled and were not reconciled for some 20 years. It is believed that the disagreement was sparked by Liston's jealousy of his protégé's success as a teacher and of his rising reputation as a surgeon.[6]

Syme was not only a gifted surgeon but was also prepared to experiment. In 1823, just starting out on his surgical career, he performed an operation on the hip joint – the first of its kind in Scotland. The patient, 19-year-old William Fraser, survived the operation without anaesthesia, but died 10 weeks later – long enough for Syme to receive general acclaim for the surgical technique.

Five years later Syme acquired even greater fame for removing a four-and-a-half pound tumour from the lower jaw of Robert Penman, an operation that Liston had refused to do because of its complexities. The patient was placed upright in a chair to prevent his blood from choking him to death and within 24 minutes the surgery was complete. Syme wrote:

> ... all this time was not employed in cutting, as I frequently allowed a little respite, to prevent exhaustion from continued suffering. The patient bore it well, and did not lose more than seven or eight ounces of blood. His breathing was never in the slightest degree affected.[7]

Despite the prominence Syme had achieved, his first application for a position at the Royal Infirmary of Edinburgh was turned down. The reason was clear – Liston was already a consultant surgeon there and managers feared repercussions from their feud.[8] But Syme, undaunted, decided to set up his own private hospital in what is now Chambers Street. Liston tried to undermine his fundraising efforts for the hospital, urging people not to lend support to 'quackery and humbug'.[9] On learning of this, Syme immediately raised an action for damages, which was only withdrawn when Liston wrote a letter of apology.

Minto House Hospital, opened in 1829 with 24 beds, an operating theatre and a lecture theatre, was run as a surgical charity and school of clinical instruction. Syme's approach of enabling students to study patients on the ward prior to operations did much to revolutionise surgical teaching. His reputation grew as he carried out complex operations for aneurysms and extensive resections of bone tumours of the upper and lower jaw. He was also possibly the first surgeon to perform a total excision of the tongue for cancer.

Syme had run Minto House Hospital for just four years when, in 1833, he was appointed Professor of Clinical Surgery at the University with a salary of £100 a year, beating Liston to the post. The appointment allowed him to care for surgical patients within the infirmary, but he had to pay a stipend of £300 a year to the previous incumbent, James Russell, the first Professor of Clinical Surgery at Edinburgh, who had held the reins for more than three decades. Syme did not have to pay up for long however, as Russell died three years later at the age of 83.[10]

When Liston left in 1835 to become Professor of Clinical Surgery at University College Hospital, London, Syme finally became the leading consulting surgeon in Scotland. At a time when the operating room was like a theatre with an audience of students, many surgeons played to the crowd. But it was Syme's skill as a surgeon rather than showmanship that enthralled. One of his colleagues, Dr Joseph Bell, recounted that

> … his operating was entirely devoid of flourish and dash… He was not rapid, not very elegant. But on the other hand, he was absolutely free from fuss and flurry… He thought of nothing but the patient, and the best – not the most rapid, not the showiest, not the easiest – but the *best* way of relieving him.[11]

In 1842 Syme was the first surgeon to carry out an amputation at the ankle – previously amputation would have been made at the thigh. The procedure, which is still called 'Syme's ankle disarticulation', made it a lot easier for the patient to walk afterwards with a prosthesis.

Syme spent virtually all his career in Edinburgh. However, when Liston died in 1847, he took up his post at University College Hospital, London, but he stayed in the city only five months before falling out with his southern colleagues and returning once again to the Chair of Clinical Surgery in Edinburgh. Syme continued to practise in Edinburgh until he suffered a stroke in 1869 and resigned his Chair.

James Young Simpson, who discovered the anaesthetic powers of chloroform, was one of Syme's contemporaries. Yet while Syme's work as a surgeon was revolutionised by the development of anaesthesia, the pair clashed on numerous occasions and when Simpson applied for the Chair of Midwifery in Edinburgh, Syme supported his main rival instead.

Simpson's background was very different from Syme's. He was born in the market town of Bathgate, 18 miles from Edinburgh. It would seem that his humble origins could have jeopardised his career: when the Town Council voted some years later on who should succeed to the Chair of Midwifery, concerns were raised that 'a poor baker's son' would be elected.[12]

Some of Simpson's critics commented that 'he was always in a hurry'; even his birth was recorded as 'born before arrival'.[13] But while he may have been in a rush to enter the world he was the last of his siblings to do so, being the eighth child and seventh son of Mary and David Simpson. A 'rosy bairn wi' laughin' mou' and dimpled cheeks',[14] he was by all accounts doted upon by his family.

When Simpson came into the world the family fortunes were not in good shape. The doctor's fee for his birth was 10 shillings; takings from the bakery the day before were just 8s 3d.[15] The income from the bakery did improve and the family moved to a better house across the street. Many thought having a seventh son had brought good fortune, but the turnaround was probably more due to Simpson's mother, Mary, taking an active role in the running of the business.

Simpson's headmaster described him as 'the wise wean', noting a lively, alert eye in the rather mature, though plump face.[16] His leaning towards medicine may have been inspired by his grandfather, Alexander Simpson, a farmer and farrier known for his ability to treat animal diseases, using both orthodox methods and those resting on superstition – he was reputed to have once helped bury a healthy cow alive in order to stop the spread of cattle plague.

Simpson's family encouraged him in his studies, hoping that one day he would go to university. This he did, arriving in Edinburgh, aged 14, wearing his brother's corduroy suit.[17] He must have excelled, for he won a £10 bursary for his Latin prose and with these much-needed funds embarked upon his second year as a student, having taken the decision to go into medicine.

Simpson demonstrated the diligent application essential for success. At his lodgings, alongside John Reid, a friend from Bathgate, Simpson got up early to cram in a few hours' study before an 8am class. The landlord, Dr McArthur, a former teacher at their Bathgate School, wrote, 'I can now do with four hours' sleep, John Reid can do with six but I have not been able to break in James yet.'[18]

As well as his compulsory University courses, Simpson took some extra-mural classes. Like Syme, who was 12 years his senior, he attended Liston's lectures. During one of these, as Liston prepared to amputate a woman's breast, the horrified look on the patient's face as the knife was about to be inserted caused Simpson to flee, declaring that he was going to study Law. Later in life he said that at that moment he had asked himself, 'Can nothing be done to make operations less painful?'[19] This may have been a crucial moment in turning him to his quest to revolutionise pain relief. Simpson could easily have ended up in obscurity. He had completed his exams for the Licentiate of the Royal College of Surgeons of Edinburgh shortly before his 19th birthday in 1830. Still too young to complete his MD, he applied for a post as a doctor at the village of Inverkip on the River Clyde. He later reflected:

When not selected, I felt perhaps a deeper amount of chagrin and disappointment than I have ever experienced since that date. If chosen, I would probably have been working there as a village doctor still.[20]

His brother John then wrote to their cousin Walter Grindlay in Liverpool, who had interests in shipping, seeking a post for him as a ship's doctor. By the time a position was found aboard *The Betsy*, in 1832, Simpson had established himself as a lecturer in Pathology.[21]

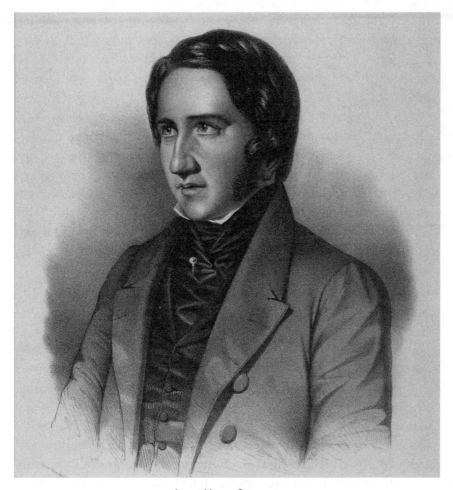

James Young Simpson.

Where fate had spared Simpson from obscurity as a village GP and from peril on the high seas, it introduced him to John Thomson, the University's first Professor of Pathology (and previously Professor of Military Surgery). To complete his MD, Simpson submitted a thesis entitled *Death from Inflammation*; he was examined by Thomson, who was so impressed that he offered him a job as his assistant.

Unlike Syme, a vociferous campaigner against Pathology as a specialty who called for its Chair to be abolished, Simpson was a staunch advocate of this way of understanding disease, especially since technical improvements to the microscope had opened up new potential for research. But for some reason Thomson encouraged him to turn his attention to midwifery. Simpson later admitted that he tended to fall asleep during midwifery lectures. Nevertheless, the Professor of Midwifery, James Hamilton, saw something special in his student and he would prove to be a major influence on Simpson's career path.

Simpson, hungry for knowledge, decided to further his medical education by visiting hospitals in Europe. Financed by one of his brothers, he travelled to Paris, Brussels, Liège, and Antwerp. On his return he was elected President of the Royal Medical Society in Edinburgh, a much coveted position among up-and-coming postgraduates.[22] He knew that all eyes would be upon him as he delivered his inaugural address, 'Diseases of the Placenta', but while he may have been nervous about public speaking, he was thorough and detailed in his research. His hard work paid off. The address received great acclaim and was later published in the *Edinburgh Medical Journal* before being translated into French, German and Italian.

Simpson was made Deputy Professor of Pathology after Thomson became ill but, as the choice of his inaugural lecture reflects, he was already more focused on obstetrics. The field of midwifery was exciting and changing rapidly. While '*accoucheurs*' – male midwives – had become fashionable in France in the 17th century, it was not until nearly a century later that this trend reached Britain, and some still considered the idea of a man being present at a birth abhorrent. In 1736 Edinburgh became the first university to have a Chair of Midwifery, but not until 1833 did the subject became compulsory for all medical students in Scotland; England followed suit 33 years later, reflecting the growing demand by more informed women for improved standards of care.[23]

Simpson's decision to pursue a career in this field represented a risk. He set up a private clinic to bring in income, gave extra-mural lectures in midwifery and worked at the Lying-In Hospital founded by Hamilton to gain more experience. He worked very long hours, but when time allowed he was an enthusiastic participant in social gatherings around the city. His convivial spirit comes across from a note jotted on the back of a visiting card:

> Dr Simpson with great regret,
> Finds himself so much beset,
> With sickly dead and dying,
> As almost sets his eyes a-crying,
> Hence ye of number 23,
> Pray don't wait for him at tea.[24]

In 1839 Hamilton resigned, leaving the Chair of Midwifery vacant. The position was allocated by Town Council vote. Despite Simpson's growing reputation it was not a foregone conclusion that he would be given the Chair. His main disadvantage was not so much his youth – he was still only 28 – but the fact that he was unmarried. The latter issue was soon rectified. In the midst of election canvassing he slipped away and on Boxing Day 1839 he married Jessie Grindlay, Walter's daughter, returning to Edinburgh immediately to continue his campaign. It was a close call, with 17 votes to 16, but Simpson won. His private practice prospered as women clamoured to be seen by this innovative young professor, who would try out new treatments rather than rely on traditional remedies such as blood-letting with leeches. Simpson's standing was also enhanced by the fact that he treated Princess Marie of Baden, wife of the Duke of Hamilton, during her confinement. As Professor of Midwifery, he refined the obstetric forceps, introducing a design that is still in use. Inspired by boys playing 'suckers' in Princes Street Gardens, he also experimented with a vacuum extractor to assist in the birthing process.[25]

Pain Relief – Defying Nature?

In 1847 Simpson started using ether to relieve the pain of women in childbirth. This followed reports that John Warren, a surgeon at the Massachusetts General Hospital, Boston, USA, had enlisted a dentist, William Morton, to help administer ether to a patient before removing a tumour from the patient's neck. Liston, at University College Hospital, London, was the first surgeon in Britain to operate using ether as an anaesthetic, during a leg amputation on a butler called Frederick Churchill.

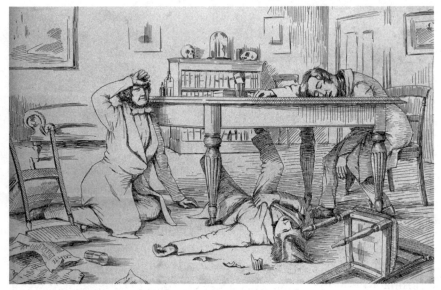

Cartoon of James Young Simpson and colleagues experimenting with chloroform.

Simpson was keen to find out more and spent his Christmas holiday with Liston. On his return to Edinburgh he was ready to try ether as an anaesthetic. Aware of its side-effects, particularly nausea and vomiting, he created an inhaler to make it easier to administer, but he was convinced there must be better anaesthetics to be had. Determined to find them, he ordered chemicals from the University Chemistry laboratory with the intention of testing them out on himself by breathing in their odours. The Professor of Chemistry, Lord Playfair, insisted he should first administer one of the substances he had amassed to two rabbits. It was fortunate he did, for both rabbits died.[26]

One November night in 1847 Simpson performed his famous experiment with chloroform in his dining room with his assistants, Dr Matthew Duncan and Dr George Keith, having learned about chloroform as a possible anaesthetic agent from David Waldie, a Liverpool chemist who qualified as a doctor in Edinburgh. The effects of its inhalation were startling. Simpson awoke to find himself on the floor. Duncan was beneath a chair unconscious and snoring, Keith was kicking the legs of the supper table. Inhalations were repeated on numerous occasions until the early hours when Simpson's niece by marriage, Agnes Petrie, took up the challenge and tried it out. A rather rotund lady, she was heard to say as she went under, 'I'm an angel, oh, an angel.'[27]

Convinced that he had found the substance he had been searching for, Simpson used chloroform successfully a few days later on a patient, Jane Carstairs, who gave birth to a baby girl called Wilhelmina. The use of anaesthesia to dull the pain of childbirth was highly controversial. Opponents argued that according to Genesis 3:16, 'In sorrow thou shalt bring forth children'. Simpson countered that, according to the Hebrew texts, 'sorrow' here meant toil or labour and not pain.[28] In 1853 the use of chloroform as an anaesthetic in childbirth gained high-profile support when it was administered both to Queen Victoria for the birth of her ninth child, Prince Leopold, and to the daughter of the Archbishop of Canterbury.[29]

Simpson received full recognition for his discovery during his lifetime and in 1866 became the first person to be knighted for services to medicine. He died at the age of 50 and although his family declined the offer of a burial site in Westminster Abbey in preference for Warriston Cemetery in Edinburgh, there is a memorial bust of him in the Abbey and a statue in Edinburgh's Princes Street Gardens to commemorate his contribution to clinical medicine.

The Father of Modern Antisepsis

While Simpson's work in anaesthesia provided much-needed pain relief, it did little to solve the problem of post-operative infection. The very fact that operations did not need to be performed as quickly meant there was more time for microbes to infect the patient and post-operative mortality rates rose. Sepsis was commonplace and surgical wards were filled with the stench of decaying flesh. Simpson himself once commented that 'the man laid on an operating table in one of our surgical wards is exposed to more chances of death than was the English soldier in the field of Waterloo'.[30] Joseph Lister was the man to address this problem. He had been strongly influenced by his time at Edinburgh Medical School, where Syme became not only his mentor but also his father-in-law. Simpson was not a supporter of Lister, perhaps because of his association with his old antagonist, Syme.

Lister was an earnest young Quaker from Essex, who was known to stutter when nervous. He completed his medical degree at University College, London (UCL), where as a student he attended the first administration of ether by Liston. Once qualified, he decided not to seek a career in surgery straight away but to further his medical education in Edinburgh. He only intended to stay a month but ended up staying seven years, not least because of the patronage of Syme.

When the 25-year-old Lister arrived in Edinburgh in 1853 he carried a letter of introduction to Syme provided by his former teacher at UCL, Professor William Sharpey, Britain's first Professor of Physiology. Although Syme had a reputation for being unapproachable and gruff, Lister was invited to dine with him when he first went to call. This warm reception was followed by the offer of a post as a clerk in Syme's operating rooms. While such a position was very junior for someone who was already a fellow of the Royal College of Surgeons in London, Lister was aware of Syme's reputation and knew that it would be a great learning experience. Syme arranged for him to carry out surgical duties at the Royal Infirmary, where the young doctor was impressed with the 200 surgical beds compared with about 60 at University College Hospital, London.[31] Lister soon became Syme's house surgeon.

A year later the dual post of Assistant Surgeon at the Royal Infirmary and Lecturer at the Royal College of Surgeons became free (the previous incumbent, a Richard Mackenzie, who had been tipped as Syme's successor, had gone to tend the wounded in the Crimea, where he had died of cholera). Lister wrote diffidently to his father:

> The question now is, should I not take advantage of this unrivalled opportunity of advancing in my profession? It is true it must depend entirely on myself (under the blessing, if I may humbly say so, of Almighty God in Christ Jesus) whether I succeed or not; but I am encouraged to hope that though I must not expect to be a Liston or a Syme still I shall get on.[32]

Lister had already taken up a role as an extra-mural lecturer, coincidentally renting the rooms formerly used by Mackenzie in High

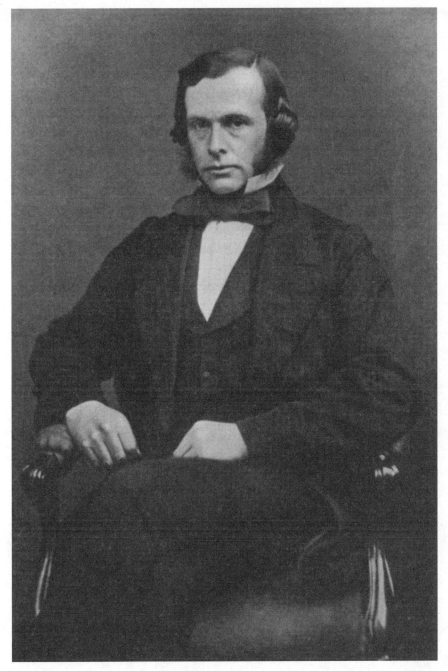

Joseph Lister.

School Yards, and had opened a consulting room at Rutland Street in Edinburgh's West End. His concerns about being appointed to Mackenzie's post proved unfounded. He got the post and in autumn 1856 was promoted to Assistant Surgeon at the Royal Infirmary of Edinburgh. A frequent visitor to Syme's home in Morningside, he started courting Syme's daughter, Agnes, and the pair married in 1856. While their honeymoon included a trip to the Lake District, much of it was spent travelling around foreign medical schools. In Pavia, Professor Porta, who held the Chair of Anatomy, proudly showed them the preserved head, forefingers and thumbs of his predecessor, Professor Antonio Scarpa, a celebrated surgeon.[33] Agnes, her father's daughter, did not flinch. Throughout their marriage, she took down her husband's lectures and notes and aided him in his work wherever possible. She wrote:

> Joseph's dictating was really wonderful – keeping me writing as fast as I possibly could, and the sentences flowing out so smoothly, hardly a word having to be altered.[34]

It was not only Agnes who showed such strong commitment. Lister had to give up being a Quaker to marry her, as the Society of Friends frowned upon marriage outside their faith. He even ordered a new door plaque, which instead of 'Joseph Lister' referred to him as 'Mr Lister', thereby rejecting the Quaker policy of not adopting titles.[35]

In 1860 Lister left Edinburgh to take the Chair in Surgery at the Royal Infirmary in Glasgow. Unlike Edinburgh, where the Chair of Surgery entitled its holder to a hospital appointment, it was more than a year before Lister was placed in charge of wards at Glasgow Royal Infirmary. In the interim he used his time to maximum effect, designing surgical instruments. These included a needle for the silver wire used to stitch wounds, a hook for the removal of peas, beads and other objects from the ear, scissors with blunt probe-shaped points for cutting a bandage or stitch so as not to prick the patient and slender forceps for entering narrow sinuses.[36]

Lister was taken aback by the conditions he encountered on the Glasgow wards. While the Edinburgh wards were far from sterile,

Syme insisted on cleanliness at operations in a bid to reduce infection. In Glasgow it was a different matter. Nobody took responsibility for hygiene and members of the lay committee in charge of cleanliness in the operating theatre were intent only on keeping costs down.[37]

Among surgeons handwashing was a rarity; many wore their blood-splattered operating aprons around the wards with evident pride and surgical instruments were given the most meagre wash between operations. At the time most people subscribed to the miasma or 'bad air' theory, which held that epidemics resulted from inhaling noxious vapours arising from swamps and rotting material. Some argued that the only way to prevent infection was to tear down the hospital buildings and have them rebuilt;[38] others believed that certain infections were part of the healing process and extolled the virtues of 'laudable' pus.

It was in this context that Lister was inspired by the work of Louis Pasteur in Paris. In the 1850s Pasteur had proved that fermentation, or rotting, was not a chemical process but was caused by living germs in the air, since it did not occur if the germs were killed by heat or excluded by air filtration. Lister drew obvious parallels with wound sepsis, but being unable to kill germs in wounds using heat as Pasteur had done in his test tubes, he set out to find a chemical substance that would have the same effect. The chemical in question turned out to be carbolic acid. After reading a newspaper article about this substance, also known as 'German creosote', being used to purify sewage at Carlisle in the north of England, Lister then used it to douse surgical instruments, wounds and dressings and produced a striking reduction in the incidence of post-operative gangrene. He published his results in a series of articles in *The Lancet* in 1867, all under the title 'On a New Method of Treating Compound Fractures, Abcesses, etc, with Observations on the Conditions of Suppuration', after which he presented his findings at a British Medical Association Meeting in Dublin, in a paper entitled 'Antiseptic Principle of the Practice of Surgery'.[39]

The specific case that put Lister's antiseptic method in the spotlight was that of James Greenlees, an 11-year-old boy who had suffered a compound fracture of his left leg when run over by a cart. His treatment involved applying undiluted carbolic acid to the wound; the dressing, soaked in the same substance, was then covered in a sheet of tinfoil to prevent evaporation. After four days there was no sign of blood-poisoning or fever and after six weeks the boy was walking without a splint. Further cases of compound fractures and other ailments were treated with equal success. Lister set about refining his antiseptic method. He discovered that carbolic acid worked just as well if diluted and found that a mixture of paraffin wax, olive oil and carbolic acid spread thinly on a calico dressing gave better results and lessened irritation.

Despite his success in reducing infection rates, many surgeons failed to appreciate Lister's revolutionary approach. It met with an apathetic response in London and in some quarters his methods were treated as quackery. There were also claims that he was not the first to promote the use of carbolic acid in medicine – which held some truth, except that hitherto its application had been haphazard.

One of Lister's severest critics was Simpson, who attacked him under the pen-name 'Chirurgicus' in the *Edinburgh Daily Review*; the piece, also reprinted in the *Lancet*, stated that Lister should not be credited with introducing carbolic acid because the Parisian doctor Jules Lemaire had previously advocated its use in medical and veterinary practice.[40] Such a criticism was missing the point – it was not so much that Lister was using carbolic acid; it was the fact that he used it in a methodical and revolutionary way to prevent infection.

Lister was philosophical, commenting that it was not the first time he had been misunderstood. He was keen to widen the use of his antiseptic methods and to do this he felt that he needed to return to London. In 1866 he applied for the Chair of Surgery at University College, London,[41] but was unsuccessful. Three years later Syme suffered a stroke and Lister was offered the Chair of Clinical Surgery at Edinburgh. This appointment came with the backing of Edinburgh students, who had petitioned him to become a candidate:

We believe, that your researches in various departments of science and your contributions to its literature have caused your name to stand next to Mr Syme amongst the living surgeons of Scotland. Your method of antiseptic treatment constitutes a well-marked epoch in the history of British surgery and will result in lasting glory to the profession and unspeakable benefit to mankind. We feel sure also that if you are appointed to this chair the benevolence of your character and the urbanity of your manners will speedily draw around you a large band of attached and devoted followers.[42]

Lister's departure from Glasgow was mired in controversy due to the publication of 'Effects of the Antiseptic System of Treatment upon the Salubrity of a Surgical Hospital', a paper in which he illustrated the efficacy of his antiseptic methods notwithstanding the proximity to his wards of burial pits used during an 1849 cholera epidemic. This was interpreted as criticism of the cleanliness of the wards although it was meant to show the success of his antiseptic methods.[43]

Back in Edinburgh, Lister would visit the Infirmary each Sunday and – in keeping with the Sabbath – went on foot so as not to employ the coachmen and horses.[44] His research focused on trying to grow the germs. The presence of such germs was ridiculed by John Hughes Bennett, an expert with the microscope famous for his description of leukaemia. Bennett regarded microbes as 'mythical fungi'.[45] 'Where are the germs?' he demanded. 'Show them to us and we will believe. Has anyone seen these germs?'[46]

Undaunted in his conviction that germs were airborne, Lister invented a carbolic acid spraying device to sterilise the air in the operating theatre, but it was so arduous to operate that one house dresser fainted from the effort.[47] The first version was improved with the addition of a long pump handle, then a steam-operated spray was introduced in 1871.[48] But Lister was not convinced about the efficacy of spraying, which caused the hands of those operating the pump to become white and was responsible for cases – mainly mild – of carbolic poisoning. After he abandoned its use, he wrote, 'As regards the spray, I feel ashamed that I should have ever recommended it for the purpose of destroying microbes in the air.'[49]

His work had received acclaim abroad, particularly in Germany, for saving many lives in the Franco–Prussian war, but Lister still had to convince surgeons in London of its value. With this in mind, he left Edinburgh in 1877 to become Professor of Surgery at King's College Hospital. Compared with his lectures in Edinburgh, which attracted up to 500 students, he struggled to pull in a crowd and when he used antiseptics on a man with a broken kneecap, one London surgeon poured scorn on his efforts: 'When this poor fellow dies someone should charge him [Lister] with not treating him properly.'[50]

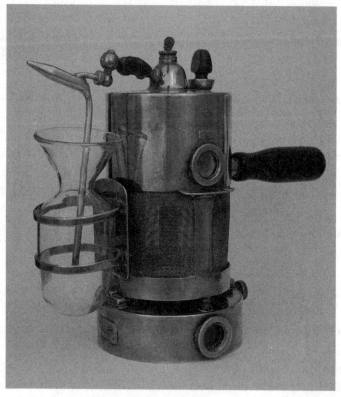

A steam-operated carbolic spraying device used in operating theatres in the 19th century.

Eventually his perseverance paid off, the virtues of his antiseptic methods were acknowledged and he became so renowned for his life-saving innovation that in 1883 he was made a Baronet. Almost a decade later, the death of his devoted wife shook Lister so much that he gave up all his research. However he was appointed President of the

Royal Society and held this position between 1895 and 1900. On his death at the age of 84, Westminster Abbey was filled with mourners. Subsequently a monument in his honour was erected in London's Portland Place. Lister's contribution to microbiology is also recognised by the naming of a bacterium after him: *Listeria monocytogenes*, which can cause listeriosis, a severe infection in the unborn child.

CHAPTER 3

Plague and Pestilence
The Dawning of Public Health

WHEN THE UNIVERSITY of Edinburgh Medical School opened its doors in 1726 the city was a very unhealthy place to live. For many centuries the Scots had suffered disproportionately from poverty, famine and destitution compared with their southern neighbours, and the burghers of Edinburgh in particular suffered from severe overcrowding which inevitably spawned disease.

In contrast, 12th and 13th century Edinburgh must have been a pleasant and well organised city. The 2,000 inhabitants living in and around the Royal Mile and the associated wynds had gardens and orchards to the rear and access to fields beyond, where cattle could graze. A surrounding wall protected them from English invasion, food was provided by local farming villages and processed by the mills of Dean Village, and there were easy trading links to Europe through the port of Leith. But as the population grew, reaching 20,000 by the time Edinburgh was proclaimed capital of Scotland in 1450, the city's limited number of dwellings had become woefully inadequate. The city's boundaries remained virtually unchanged for 600 years. Favoured options for extra living space included building in the garden areas, thus obliterating most of the town's green spaces, and extending the upper storeys of existing houses with timber balconies projecting over the narrow streets and wynds, blocking out fresh air and sunlight. When these efforts failed to accommodate the burgeoning population there was only one way to go, and that was up. Tenement buildings in the Old Town grew taller and more cramped year by year until no one knew exactly where everyone lived except the 'water caddies' – men and women who carried water from street pumps in barrels on their backs up the dark and narrow staircases to sell the contents for a penny a barrel to the rich families inhabiting the comparatively light and airy upper storeys. Inevitably the combination of poverty and overcrowding, the lack of sanitation and fresh air, and an inadequate diet led to poor health. Infectious diseases were the leading cause of death for several centuries and epidemics were rife, with plague, smallpox and typhus fever being the major killers.

Although most doctors recognised the contagious nature of diseases like smallpox, measles and scarlet fever, they believed that they were spread by foul smells and noxious vapours, which must have been plentiful in 17th and 18th century Edinburgh, and this coloured their thinking about prevention and control measures.

The Plague

The plague first arrived in Edinburgh in 1349 as the Black Death spread inexorably from the south. Characterised by buboes – huge swelling of the lymph glands – human epidemics take hold only after outbreaks among house (black) rats. These animals die rapidly of the disease, leaving their starving, microbe-carrying fleas to turn to human blood for sustenance, thereby sparking an epidemic. In 14th century Edinburgh each household would have hosted its own rat colony.

There is virtually no information on the death toll from the Black Death in Edinburgh, or in Scotland as a whole, but in London it killed an estimated 40 per cent of the population. According to the chronicler John of Fordun, an Edinburgh resident who lived through the pandemic:

There was, in the kingdom of Scotland so great a pestilence and plague among men... as from the beginning of the world even unto modern times, had never been heard of by man, nor is found in books, for the enlightenment of those who come after. For, to such a pitch did that plague wreak its cruel spite, that nearly a third of mankind were thereby made to pay the debt of nature. Moreover, by God's will, this evil led to a strange and unwonted kind of death, insomuch that the flesh of the sick was somehow puffed out and swollen, and they dragged out their earthly life for barely two days... Men shrank from it so much that, through fear of contagion, sons, fleeing as from the face of leprosy or from an adder, durst not go and see their parents in the throes of death.[1]

After the Black Death the plague continued to visit Edinburgh at intervals for nearly 300 years. During epidemics the sick were deposited in wooden huts built on Holyrood Park and Burgh Muir, a moor to the south of the city which includes present-day Bruntsfield Links, while those who had been in contact with cases were isolated and their houses fumigated with burning whin, heather and straw.[2] On occasions Inchkeith and other islands in the Firth of Forth were used as quarantine stations.[3] A particularly severe epidemic in 1568–69, dubbed the Great Plague of Edinburgh and said to have been carried into the city by a merchant, killed 2,500 citizens. The symptoms were described as:

sowning [swooning], cold sweats, vomiting; excrements corrupt, teuch [tough]; urine black, or colour of lead. Cramps, convulsion of limbs, imperfection of speech and stinking breath, colic, swelling of the body as in dropsy, visage of divers colours, God's token [red spots] quickly discovered and covering themselves.[4]

The final plague epidemic in Edinburgh in 1645 was so severe that 'scarce 60 men were left capable of assisting in its [the city's] defence'.[5] Indeed during the outbreak the University moved to Linlithgow. Although there are no mortality rates for Edinburgh, records show that 60 per cent of the people of Leith succumbed.[6]

Smallpox

Smallpox was another deadly infection that visited the city regularly from the 16th century until it was prevented by widespread vaccination

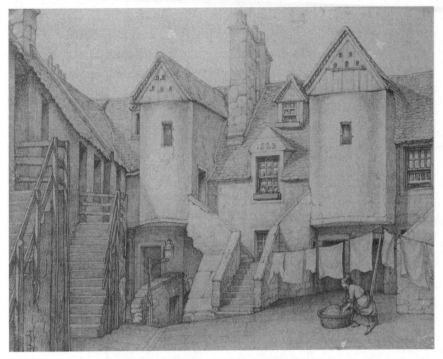

Tenement building in White Horse Close.

in the mid-19th century. Perhaps the most dreaded of all epidemic diseases, it appeared unannounced, mainly striking infants and young children. It killed around 20 per cent of those it infected and scarred and even blinded many of the survivors. Records from Edinburgh in the 18th century show that smallpox was the commonest cause of death in early childhood: it accounted for one in 10 of all deaths and during a severe outbreak in 1740–42 this figure rose to 17 per cent. The symptoms included high fever, extremely painful, suppurating throat ulcers and the characteristic skin pocks. The airborne virus spreads best in cramped and airless conditions typical of the dwellings of the poor.

Smallpox inoculation reached Scotland in 1726, after its introduction to London in 1721 by Lady Mary Wortley Montague, wife of the British ambassador to the Ottoman Empire. She first saw the ancient custom of inoculation used to prevent smallpox in Constantinople and, having suffered from the disease herself, was keen to protect others. The practice involved transferring the infection from one person to another by scratching the skin with a needle containing a small dose of live virus taken from the pock of a victim. This generally caused a mild illness with a few pocks and resulted in long-term immunity. Although it carried a 1–2 per cent risk of causing full-blown smallpox, inoculation saved many lives prior to the introduction of Edward Jenner's cowpox vaccination in the early 1800s. Initial uptake in Scotland was patchy, with city dwellers and the upper classes more enthusiastic than the poor and country folk. Many had religious objections to its use. Sir John Sinclair, editor of *Statistical Account of Scotland* from 1791–99, observed:

> Multitudes of the common people considered inoculation as criminal; – as an encroachment upon the prerogative of Providence; as tempting Providence; – as implying an impious distrust of Divine Providence, and a vain attempt to alter His irreversible decrees.[7]

The Fever

Like smallpox, 'the fever' was a constant visitor to the tenements of Edinburgh. The term covered a variety of infections, but typhus spread by body lice, and typhoid, mainly acquired through drinking contaminated water, were the biggest killers. The microbes causing these lethal infections thrived among the poor and destitute in their crowded, unhygienic homes and continued unabated until the public health measures of the 19th century finally improved the lot of the poor.

In 18th century Edinburgh the situation deteriorated as the population grew. By 1740 the city had 50,000 inhabitants with an estimated 10 per cent occupying dwellings in streets, 60 per cent in closes and 20 per cent in dugouts, sheds and the like; 10 per cent were vagrants.[8] In 1700 a 14-storey building on the Royal Mile, aptly named Babylon, collapsed in flames and, in 1751, when another old house collapsed, a building survey indicated that many tenements were in a similarly dangerous state of disrepair.

The death rate in Edinburgh fell between 1740 and 1820 as a result of the migration of the wealthy to the New Town, but this also opened a geographical as well as a social gulf, which made it easier for the rich to ignore the plight of the poor. An influx of country folk in search of work soon filled the space vacated in the Old Town and there was a return to severe overcrowding, with Edinburgh's total population topping 100,000 by 1800. A large contingent of labourers, many escaping famine in Ireland, began arriving in 1818 to build the Union Canal, work in the new steam-powered industries, and later to construct the 'Innocent Railway' running from Dalkeith to Edinburgh. These immigrant labourers were particularly vulnerable to diseases that were endemic in the common lodging houses in the Old Town. It was said that:

> A lodger fresh from the country often lies down in a bed filled with infection by its last tenant, or from which the corpse of a victim to fever has only been removed a few hours before.[9]

It is no wonder that these unfortunates filled the wards of the Royal Infirmary. Visitors to the Old Town were appalled, one writing:

> I never came to my own lodging in Edenborough, or went out, but I was constrained to hold my nose, or to use wormwood, or some such scented plant.[10]

Author Tobias Smollett complained of the 'stercoraceous' odours, and James Boswell, recording Samuel Johnson's visit to the capital in 1773, recorded in his diary: 'A zealous Scotsman would have wished Mr Johnson to be without one of his five senses upon this occasion.'[11]

Cholera

Cholera hit the UK for the first time in 1830 and arrived in Edinburgh in 1831, with further epidemics in 1838, 1848–49 and 1853–54. Each caused alarm and panic as healthy people were struck down with diarrhoea and vomiting so severe that they could die from dehydration within 48 hours. Mainly spread by sewage contamination of drinking water, this bacterium easily invaded a city where safe drinking water was at a premium. The first epidemic killed 1,065 people. Since the late 17th century the Old Town water supply had been piped from a spring in the village of Comiston to a reservoir on Castle Hill, and from there to six wells along the Royal Mile. But as the population grew this arrangement became increasingly inadequate despite additional supplies from springs in the villages of Liberton and Swanston. In 1824 a reservoir at Glencorse in the Pentland Hills was built, which provided a plentiful supply.[12] However, with the simultaneous piping of water to all the buildings in the New Town, Old Town dwellers were obliged to queue at stand-pipes for their water. This was then stored in their filthy dwellings – a recipe for the spread of infection.

The 1832 cholera epidemic in London gave reformers such as Edwin Chadwick, a great believer in the miasma theory of contagion, the impetus to begin the clean-up with the installation of new water and sewage systems. In Edinburgh too, the rapid spread of cholera was widely acknowledged to have been caused by conditions in the Old Town. The Royal College of Physicians called for more stand-pipes, for privies and WCs to be installed in houses, for the closes to be cleaned up and paved, and for there to be increased access to light, air and water, and regular waste collections. But although the Town Council made some progress in implementing these changes, it was not enough to prevent further cholera epidemics.

Death rates in Edinburgh rose during the 1830s and 1840s. In 1845 Dr James Stark, Registrar of Mortality of Edinburgh and Leith, calculated for the first time the annual death rates separately for each social class. The message was clear: by far the highest death rates were among the lowest classes (labourers, porters and paupers). Just over seven per cent of deaths among the higher and wealthier classes occurred in babies under the age of one, but this increased to more than 24 per cent in the lowest classes. In the highest class the average lifespan was 47 years, compared with 26 in the lowest.[13]

Two years later Stark published a damning report entitled *Inquiry into Some Points of the Sanitary State of Edinburgh*.[14] The drainage system in Edinburgh's Old Town was at best rudimentary, if not non-existent. For several centuries a system of open sewers, aptly named 'foul burns', had drained the streets, either into natural water-courses or into irrigated meadows where it was used to fertilise the pastures. These meadows, mainly situated outwith the city at Craigentinny, Lochend and Dalry, were described by the police commissioners thus:

> These rank and fetid exhalations poison the air for miles around. They are insufferable to passengers, and to those living in the neighbourhood. They are carried by the wind into the City – into the Palace – and into the barracks; and after being condensed in the atmosphere by the evening's cold, they fall down in the form of damps, bringing with them sickness and disease.[15]

Stark's report led to the installation of three more open sewers, but these were still not connected to buildings. The idea was that excess water from stand-pipes would flush waste from the filthy closes into these and other water channels around the city, but in practice there was too little water for the system to work effectively. The controversy continued for more than a century with medical men unable to convince the Town Council that the sewers were a hazard to public health. Their arguments were not helped by the lack of support from the celebrated miasma theorist, Chadwick, who was not averse to the irrigation of meadows when he saw how much this increased their productivity with 'four or five crops of hay a year and supporting 4,000 milk cows'.[16] And although he did support covering the open sewers, this was not completed in Edinburgh until the beginning of the 20th century.

The Poor and Mentally Ill

Poor Laws existed in Scotland since 1579 for 'the punishment of strong and idle beggars, and relief of the poor and impotent'. In reality this was little more than the Town Council's attempt to control the hordes of beggars who frequented the streets and harassed the burghers, with the sick and infirm left to the charity of religious and voluntary bodies operating at the time. The 1579 Scottish Poor Law differed from that of England and other European countries in providing no relief for the able-bodied destitute who were generally felt to have brought

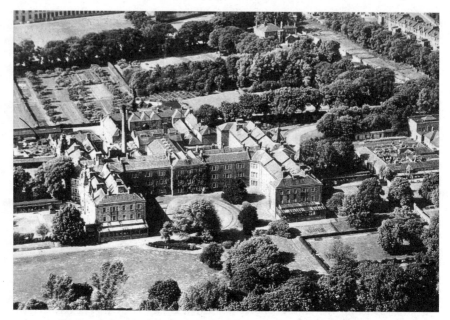

Edinburgh Lunatic Asylum, later renamed the Royal Edinburgh Hospital.

their problems on themselves by being lazy and slothful. It was perceived as morally wrong for the State to offer them support. Public health enforcement was considered a matter for the police, specifically 'medical police', to enforce and from 1771 onwards this was overseen by Boards of Police Commissioners, forerunners of the Public Health Department.

The welfare of the mentally ill, known as the insane, was also ignored by the legislation and in Edinburgh these unfortunates were generally confined in the city 'bedlam', part of the charity workhouse in Teviot Place. Here they suffered under the most atrocious conditions – confined to small, dark cells with only a pile of straw for a bed. Much needed reform to this system was instigated by Andrew Duncan, Professor of the Theory of Medicine at the University of Edinburgh. Duncan was a warm-hearted man, always concerned about the plight of the poor and chronically sick.

It is said that his interest in the care of the mentally ill was sparked by the tragic death of one of his patients, the 24-year-old poet Robert Fergusson. An inspiration to Robert Burns, who called him his 'brother in verse', Fergusson was a long-term sufferer of a manic-depressive illness and when his mother was unable to cope with an attack of 'furious insanity' there was no alternative but to send him to the bedlam where he eventually died in 1774.

Duncan was moved to launch an appeal to fund a new asylum where patients could receive care and have some hope of recovery, and in 1806 a property with four acres of land was purchased in Morningside. A royal charter was granted in 1807 and the construction of the Edinburgh Lunatic Asylum commenced in 1809. The first building, designed by architect Robert Reid and called East House, opened in 1813. This provided much improved accommodation but only for those who could pay for their keep. In 1842 West House, designed by architect William Burn, opened for the poor and in 1844 the inmates of the bedlam were transferred there. The asylum was renamed The Royal Edinburgh Hospital for Mental and Nervous Disorders in 1922, the name it retains today.

In 17th and 18th century Scotland, there is no doubt that attitudes towards the destitute delayed the instigation of public health measures similar to those being implemented in England at the time. But by the beginning of the 19th century there was a rising tide of public concern for the plight of the poor in Edinburgh, led by the foremost physicians, surgeons and ministers of the day. Prominent among these was William Pulteney Alison, Professor of Jurisprudence (later called forensic medicine, and closely linked to public health), and afterwards Professor of Medicine, at the University of Edinburgh. He graduated from the University in 1811 and in 1815 was appointed Physician to the New Town Dispensary in East Thistle Street.[17] Here he gained first-hand experience of the connection between destitution and disease. He identified lodging houses as hotbeds of infection and the wandering vagrants who frequented them as the means of spreading the diseases. In his influential pamphlet of 1840, *Observations on the Management of the Poor in Scotland and its Effect on the Health in the Great Towns*,[18] he challenged the miasma theory as being too simplistic, arguing that social factors such as overcrowding and destitution facilitated the spread of disease. He maintained that since these were not the fault of the individuals concerned, the able-bodied poor should receive state support funded through public taxes. He showed that destitution was greater in Scotland than in other European countries and that this was responsible for the increase in epidemic diseases,[19] and pressed strongly for reform of the Poor Law:

> While there has been much disposition to relieve the sick poor, there has been very general discouragement of institutions for the relief of mere poverty – of the unemployed poor, the aged or permanently disabled poor, and the widows and orphans of the poor. The whole sum applied to these purposes is much smaller than in all the English towns.[20]

It was largely due to Alison's work that the Royal Commission on the Poor Laws of Scotland was set up in 1843. In 1845 the Poor Laws were amended, although not as radically as the reformers would have liked. The duty of the community to provide relief for the poor and sick was clearly outlined, but the law fell short of addressing the massive destitution problem which remained a serious threat to the collective health of the city until Edinburgh's first Officer of Health was appointed in 1862.

In the intervening period Boards of Police Commissions continued their responsibility for public health, including lighting, cleaning, drainage and control of epidemics, as well as providing the city's police force. Many pleaded for the appointment of a Medical Officer of Health, but to no avail. The Town Council was corrupt, its inertia serving those with vested interests in opposing the much-needed changes. There was pressure from home-owners, for whom any attempt to improve the housing of the poor would mean an increase in rates, and from the millers of Dean Village and others along the Water of Leith, whose livelihood was potentially threatened by the use of the river water for sanitary improvements. The Craigentinny foul burn and its irrigated meadow, despite being the most extensive and feared of Edinburgh's sewage systems, was not covered until the early 20th century because 'the Town Council was reluctant to confront an influential landowner [the Earl of Moray], particularly while the meadows were still in full use'.[21]

It took a series of disastrous events to get agreement for the appointment of an Officer of Health. These included a major typhus outbreak in 1847 and cholera epidemics in 1848–49 and 1853–54. But the tipping-point came at 1am on Sunday 24 November 1861 when the tenement building at 99–103 High Street 'ran together with a hideous uproar and tumbled, storey upon storey, to the ground'.[22] Thirty-five people were killed in the incident and many more seriously injured. One young man lying under the debris was heard to encourage his rescuers by shouting 'Heave awa', lads, I'm no deid yet.' The incident was commemorated with a stone head of the youth set in an archway over the entrance to Paisley Close, which can still be seen today.[23] The repercussions were immense; public meetings were held, sermons preached, letters written to the press and a deputation was sent to the council, all highly critical of the lack of sanitary reform. Finally, on 30 September 1862, Police Surgeon Dr Henry Littlejohn, supported by the Presidents of the Royal Colleges of Physicians and Surgeons, Professors James Syme and James Simpson, was duly elected to the post of Medical Officer of Health for Edinburgh – the first position of its kind in Scotland.

Littlejohn, an experienced public health doctor, commanded the respect of his colleagues. A man of huge energy and foresight, and well versed in his home city's problems, he succeeded in making long overdue changes.

Born in 1826, the seventh son of Thomas Littlejohn, master baker, and Isabella Duncan of Leith Street, he attended Perth Academy and Edinburgh Royal High School, entering the University of Edinburgh to study Medicine in 1841. After he graduated in 1847 he worked as a house surgeon at Edinburgh Royal Infirmary before travelling to Paris, Vienna and Berlin to further his training. He then returned to the Royal Infirmary as Assistant Pathologist and was elected Fellow of the Royal College of Surgeons of Edinburgh in 1854.

In the same year he was appointed Police Surgeon, a part-time position answerable to the Town Council. His responsibilities included examining and treating sick policemen, prisoners and children in reformatories, as

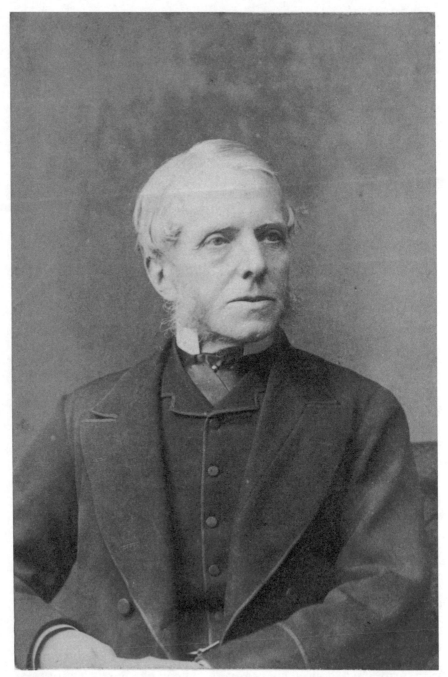

Henry Littlejohn. Photograph of by Moffat.

well as investigating sudden deaths, including murders and accidents. This marked the beginning of his career in forensic medicine and from then on he made regular appearances in the courts as medical examiner for the Crown, gaining a reputation as a fine orator and a meticulous and fair-minded medical detective.

In 1856 Littlejohn began lecturing on forensic medicine at the extra-mural medical school in Surgeon's Hall and continued to do so for 42 years. He illustrated his lectures with real live forensic cases, much appreciated by the students who packed the theatre to hear him. Among them was the young Arthur Conan Doyle, who attended the University between 1876 and 1881 and is said to have used the descriptions of Edinburgh courtroom dramas in his famous Sherlock Holmes novels.

As Edinburgh's first Medical Officer of Health, Littlejohn was installed in two rooms in the Police Chambers in the High Street with a staff of two policemen who acted as sanitary inspectors. This tiny band had a daunting task ahead but Littlejohn took it in his stride. He visited the office every morning to 'receive complaints from the inhabitants as to nuisances and sanitary defects' and then inspected the offending premises, be they tenements, bakehouses, markets or slaughterhouses.[24]

One of Littlejohn's early successes was to persuade the Lord Provost's Committee, to which he was now answerable, to pass the General Vaccination Act for Scotland in 1863. This ensured that children were vaccinated against smallpox within six months of birth, generally at a cost to the parents, but from 1867 onwards vaccination was free to all during smallpox epidemics. Defaulters were visited by an official vaccinator appointed by each Parochial Board who vaccinated the children there and then unless the parents objected. This proved to be a safe procedure; 855,185 vaccinations were performed in Scotland between 1883 and 1890 with just 22 vaccination-associated deaths.

As the number of vaccinations rose, so smallpox cases began to decline, although the disease was not completely eliminated until the 1940s. Most epidemics began in lodging houses, where one case could expose so many non-vaccinated lodgers that it was almost impossible to isolate them all during the quarantine period. Thus when there was a smallpox outbreak in 1904 Littlejohn decided to vaccinate all inmates of lodging houses, but this was only achieved after each was offered the sum of 2s 6d as an inducement. During this outbreak Littlejohn noticed that the majority of the 168 cases were adults who had been previously vaccinated, with only eight cases of children under 14 years of age. This clearly demonstrated the importance of re-vaccination after 10 years, but even so Littlejohn failed to persuade the Town Council that this should be made compulsory.

In 1865 Littlejohn presented his damning *Report on the Sanitary Conditions of Edinburgh*. At last convinced that sanitary reform was essential for the health of the city, the Town Council committed funds for the daunting task and in 1867 the Edinburgh Improvement Act and the Public Health (Scotland) Act were passed, leading to the establishment of a Public Health Committee of the Town Council in 1872. This body had a remit to control epidemics and other health hazards, run the fever hospitals and take action against owners who kept their premises in an unsanitary or dilapidated state, or without a clean water supply. At last Edinburgh was coming into line with other European cities.

From the early days of his appointment, Littlejohn realised that control of infectious disease epidemics was paramount in reducing the death rates in Edinburgh. To this end, his personal surveillance team, in the form of his two policemen, set out to identify any disease outbreak in its early stages, before the death returns indicated an epidemic. One was assigned to inspecting lodging houses, the other monitored admissions to the fever wards at the Royal Infirmary and supervised the disinfection of patients' homes when required.

Once he suspected an epidemic Littlejohn asked the city's doctors to notify him of any cases in their practice and offered help transporting the sick to hospital and disinfecting the premises. But the response was so poor that he decided that compulsory notification was the only way forward.

Despite opposition from the medical profession, he persuaded the Town Council to include the following clause in their Edinburgh Municipal and Police Act of 1879:

In order to secure more prompt action in dealing with infectious diseases, every medical practitioner practising within the burgh shall, within 24 hours of the same coming to his knowledge, report to the medical officer of health every case of cholera, typhus fever, typhoid fever, diphtheria, smallpox, scarlet fever, scarlatina, and measles... occurring in his practice, and stating the house or place where the patient is being treated, under a penalty not exceeding 40 shillings; and if it be found on inquiry by the medical officer of health that the diagnosis of such practitioner was correct, such practitioner shall be paid the sum of two shillings and six pence for each case reported...[25]

As a consequence, compulsory notification was introduced in Edinburgh in 1880, the first instance in Britain and a significant step forward. By 1882 Littlejohn reported not only its success but also its approval by the initially sceptical medical profession. In 1897 notification of infectious diseases became compulsory throughout Scotland.

During his long tenure as Medical Officer of Health, Littlejohn oversaw many improvements in the care of patients with infectious diseases and those in contact with them, not least in the hospital facilities available for their isolation and treatment. Until the 1860s infectious disease patients requiring hospitalisation were admitted to the fever wards of the Royal Infirmary and the Royal Hospital for Sick Children, but during epidemics these wards were swamped. In 1866 when a cholera epidemic threatened Edinburgh, the managers of the Royal Infirmary intimated that they would not admit any cases. In the ensuing crisis the Town Council set up temporary wards in the City Poorhouse Hospital. This situation made it clear to Littlejohn that a hospital dedicated entirely to infectious diseases was urgently needed. Consequently the Town Council bought the Canongate Poorhouse from the Parochial Board for £1,600 and converted it into the first City Fever Hospital. This opened in 1870, but as early as 1871, when a smallpox epidemic struck the city, the Royal Infirmary again refused to admit any cases. It was obvious that the new Fever Hospital was too small to cope with the number of patients. This proved to be the case

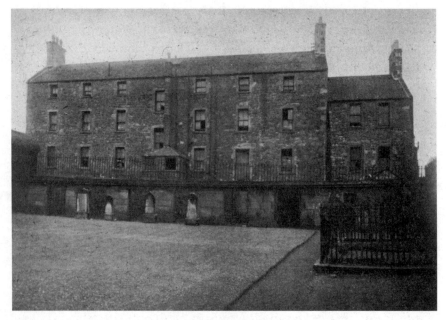

Canongate Fever Hospital.

during successive epidemics, culminating in a large outbreak of scarlet fever in 1881. Littlejohn urged the council to find a site for a new hospital, and when the Royal Infirmary moved to Lauriston Place, the council bought the old buildings in High School Yard for £28,500 and converted them into a 260-bed Fever Hospital which opened in 1885. This had isolation facilities, a 'House of Reception', where patients' close contacts could be quarantined until deemed non-infectious, and a disinfection unit that used fumes of burning sulphur until a modern steam disinfector was installed in 1905.

The conveyance of the sick to the City Fever Hospital was a problem that was solved when the Hospital Managers signed a contract with a Mrs Moir of 10–11 St James Place, who hired out an open, horse-drawn coach for patient transport; this was later replaced by a covered funeral brougham with the back removed to allow access for stretchers. She also provided transport to remove infected material from patients' homes to the disinfection unit at the Fever Hospital. In 1888 the Hospital Management Committee complained about her high prices, which she agreed to reduce to 'four shillings for the first turnout of the day, the remainder for that day will be a reduction of one shilling – that will be three shillings'.[26] Mrs Moir was still in business in 1900, by which time she was providing separate coaches for scarlet fever, diphtheria and typhoid fever cases, and had agreed to fit rubber tyres to her vehicles to provide the occupants with a more comfortable ride to hospital.[27] The first motorised ambulance was purchased in 1909.

The second City Fever Hospital also proved inadequate; in 1894 concurrent smallpox and scarlet fever epidemics far exceeded its capacity and patients had to be accommodated in hastily erected wooden huts in Holyrood Park. This fiasco prompted the council to buy a 130-acre plot at Colinton Mains, where a new 600-bed fever hospital – the third City Hospital for Infectious Diseases – was opened by Edward VII in 1903. With a later addition of another 200 beds, it served the needs of Edinburgh until the incidence of infectious diseases began to decline. From the 1960s onwards it catered for more general patients, closing in 1999 in anticipation of the opening of the New Royal Infirmary at Little France.

Tuberculosis (TB)
Just like the acute epidemic infections rife in 18th and 19th century Edinburgh, TB – also called phthisis, meaning wasting, or, more generally, consumption – thrived in the crowded, airless dwellings of the poor. But it touched all social classes. In 1888 Littlejohn wrote:

> I hardly ever open a body of a person dying of an injury or disease, but traces of the previous existence of tubercle in the lungs are found, and it is apparent that this disease has been arrested and a cure effected.[28]

But the microbe hiding in these 'cured' lung lesions could reactivate at any time causing the chronic debilitating and ultimately fatal symptoms of consumption. Although the lungs are the commonest site for the infection, the disease could also affect the lymph glands (scrofula) or the bones, particularly the spine (Pott's Disease). In addition, before the grading of milk as tuberculin-tested or pasteurised was made compulsory in 1922, most cows were infected with bovine TB which spread to humans, mostly children, through drinking infected milk.

Given the chronic nature of the disease, the pattern of TB epidemics was very different from the explosive epidemics typical of acute infections, and consequently much easier to ignore. Nevertheless it was an increasingly common killer among the children and elderly of the poor and destitute in the 17th and 18th centuries. However, the rich and famous did not escape; literary giants Emily Brontë, John Keats and Anton Chekhov all died of the disease, and in Edinburgh Robert Louis Stevenson spent some time in hospital being treated for TB of the bone by Sir Joseph Lister.

Sir Robert William Philips pioneered the care of patients with TB in Edinburgh, initiating an organised system of diagnosis, treatment, care and prevention in a career dedicated to fighting the disease. Philips was born in Aberdeen, but the family moved to Edinburgh when his father became minister of St John's Free Church. After attending the Royal High School, Philips moved on to the University of Edinburgh. He first graduated in Arts and then with honours in Medicine in 1882. In that same year, in Berlin, Robert Koch isolated the tubercle bacillus, the microbe causing TB.

After a period as house physician at Edinburgh Royal Infirmary, Philips studied in Leipzig and Vienna, seeing the tubercle bacillus under the microscope for the first time during his travels. Nowadays it is difficult to appreciate just how exciting the new 'germ theory' of infectious disease must have been. It caught Philips' imagination and by the time he returned to Edinburgh in 1883 he was determined to devote his career to the study of TB. This was despite one professor telling him, 'Don't think of such a thing. Phthisis is worn to a very thin thread. The subject is exhausted.'[29] Undaunted, he received a gold medal in 1887 for his MD thesis, *An Aetiological and Therapeutic Study of Phthisis*.

Philips began work at the New Town Dispensary in 1885. He immediately started to revolutionise the management and treatment of patients with TB. Some were treated at the Royal Infirmary and others at the city's dispensaries, but for those too poor or sick to access this care there was no help available. Philips envisaged a dispensary and hospital both dedicated entirely to the care of TB patients. Within two years he and his supporters had made this a reality. Located in three upstairs rooms at 13 Bank Street, overlooking Princes Street, it was the first specialised TB dispensary in the world. Consumptives, however poor or sick, could get the medicine and food they needed as well as advice on the benefits of fresh air and a healthy diet. Their homes were visited to trace and treat other TB sufferers, thus preventing further spread of the disease.

Within weeks of opening, the clinic was crowded with patients. In 1891 a larger clinic was opened in Lauriston Place with waiting rooms, two consulting rooms, facilities for examining the larynx, a laboratory and a dispensary. When fully established this clinic catered for around 17,000 patients a year and doctors made approximately 140 home visits each month. The bedridden were visited by volunteers who ensured that the necessary aid was provided by charitable organisations or the parish. Philips advocated fresh air for all TB sufferers and believed in the principles of rest until the healing process was under way, followed by a programme of natural movement and regular exercise to assist in the repair of muscular tissue which, he thought, had been wasted due to 'constitutional intoxication' during the active phase of the disease. He devised a series of planned walks on the Meadows, Bruntsfield Links and Arthur's Seat, which patients were encouraged to take, apparently with excellent results.[30]

In 1898 the Town Council put the following motion to the Public Health Committee:

That having regard to the opinion now maintained by leading medical men that consumption is an infectious and preventable disease, it be remitted to the Public Health Committee to consider whether any, and what, steps ought to be taken by the Local Authority to protect the public against the disease in Edinburgh, and to report.[31]

The resulting enquiry sought advice from Philips and Littlejohn, as well as the two Royal Colleges and the University Medical Faculty. Littlejohn provided figures showing that the overall mortality from TB in the city in 1899 averaged two per thousand, with the highest rates in the poorest and most crowded areas, including George Square, Broughton, the Canongate and St Giles. His recommendation was to continue the improvement policy and to distribute leaflets in poorer areas explaining the cause of TB and how to prevent it. He particularly deplored the habit of spitting which he regarded as 'not only a disgusting but a dangerous habit'.[32] Whether TB should be a notifiable disease was much debated. In the end, a policy of voluntary notification was introduced in 1903. However this did not work well and in 1907 compulsory notification was implemented.

By the late 1800s aero-therapy for TB was in vogue, pioneered by Hermann Brehmer, a doctor from Silesia who, while working in Berlin in the 1850s, was diagnosed with TB and advised by his doctor to find a healthier place to live. He travelled to the Himalayas, where his TB was cured. On returning to Berlin he wrote a thesis entitled *Tuberculosis is a Curable Disease*. He opened the first TB sanatorium in Görbersdorf in Silesia in 1863 where he advocated plenty of high altitude fresh air and a healthy diet, with encouraging results. Philips believed that this type of treatment could also be effective in Scotland and for this purpose Craigleith House, a large Georgian property in Comely Bank with extensive grounds, was acquired and converted into the Royal Victoria Hospital for Consumption. It opened in 1894. Patients were encouraged to follow Philips' programme of rest and exercise, and many stayed on as staff once they had recovered. In 1909 a farm colony, Springfield, was also set up so that cured patients could live a healthy and sheltered life away from the rigours of the city.

Thus Philips created a comprehensive scheme for TB treatment and control, centred around the dispensary where patients were either cleared for home treatment, assigned to the sanatorium and later the farm, or for advanced cases, admitted to hospital. This 'Edinburgh Scheme' was copied by many towns and cities throughout the UK and internationally. Interestingly, the first dispensary in England opened in 1909, pioneered by a group of volunteers including Edith McGaw from

Australia who later became Philips' wife.

Philips was knighted in 1913 for his achievements and was appointed to the first Chair of Tuberculosis at the University of Edinburgh in 1917. He died at the age of 82, seven years before the introduction of streptomycin for the treatment of TB in 1946; the BCG vaccination for prevention followed in 1950.

Germ Theory

Littlejohn's long career spanned the revolution in understanding the cause of infectious diseases from miasma to germs, which brought with it huge excitement, enthusiasm and optimism. As a result of the pioneering work of Louis Pasteur in Paris and Robert Koch in Berlin, the causes of anthrax, cholera, typhoid fever, diphtheria, TB and many other infections were identified in rapid succession. By the end of the 19th century there was a feeling that the epidemics of infectious diseases that had plagued the city for so long could be conquered.

Recognition of the urgent need for new diagnostic laboratories was facilitated by Pasteur's visit to Edinburgh in 1884 to attend the University's tercentenary celebrations. Pasteur's early work had been on the fermentation process, and while in Edinburgh he stayed with the Younger family and visited their brewery, where he met Alexander Low Bruce, a partner in the firm. The Bruce family, together with another brewer, Sir John Usher of Norton, were inspired to fund a Chair of Public Health, the first in Britain. Sir John also funded the University's John Usher Institute of Public Health in Warrender Park Road, where bacteriological testing was carried out.

During his 46 years in office (1862–1908), Littlejohn saw a vast improvement in the incidence of infectious disease in Edinburgh, mainly because of improvements in housing, public health awareness and early warning systems, isolation of cases and contacts and, in the case of smallpox, vaccination. Death rates fell from 26 to 14 per thousand, infant mortality from 145 to 114 per thousand, infectious diseases from six to less than one per thousand, and while the population more than doubled from 170,444 to 350,761, the population density fell from 49 to 31 people per acre.[33] Water-borne diseases such as cholera and typhoid fever, always more of a threat in the Old Town than the New, fell dramatically in the late 19th and early 20th centuries following the introduction of clean, piped water supplies. The last cholera outbreak was in 1866–67 with 391 cases and 154 deaths. Despite several alarms, not a single case has been reported in Edinburgh since. However the same cannot be said for typhoid fever, which has reappeared from time to time, most recently in 1970 when four cases were notified; three of the sufferers had drunk water from the Water of Leith and the fourth was the brother of one of these cases. The source of the infection was eventually found to be a sewage-contaminated storm drain which linked to a group of houses in which one occupant was a carrier of the microbe.[34] Similarly, with typhus fever that thrives in unhygienic, cramped surroundings, the number of notified cases dropped from 355 with 102 deaths for the period 1880–89, to 139 cases and 22 deaths between 1890 and 1899. The last reported case was in 1907.

Despite his busy life as Medical Officer of Health, Littlejohn had many other responsibilities. He was President of the Royal College of Surgeons in 1875, President of Edinburgh Medico-Chirurgical Society from 1883 to 1885 and President of the Royal Institution of Public Health in 1893. He was also Director of the Sick Children's Hospital, manager of the Royal Infirmary of Edinburgh and chairman of the Scottish Society for the Prevention of Cruelty to Children. He was knighted in 1895 for his achievements in improving the public health of the citizens of Scotland and died at his country house, Benreoch, in Arrochar, Argyll aged 88. Littlejohn was succeeded in his role as Medical Officer of Health by Alfred Maxwell Williamson, previously Chief Sanitary Inspector, and in his Chair of Forensic Medicine by his son Henry Harvey Littlejohn. Although there was still much for his successors to do in the field of public health, Littlejohn will always be acknowledged as having taken the first steps in conquering infectious disease epidemics in Edinburgh.

CHAPTER 4
Women in Medicine
Early Struggles in Edinburgh

THE FIRST WOMAN ever to qualify in medicine and practice in the UK graduated from the University of Edinburgh Medical School in 1812. Masquerading as a man, her case was definitely unique and although it did not set a precedent for the future of women in medicine, it certainly makes an intriguing story.

A student named James Barry studied medicine in Edinburgh from 1809 to 1812 and after a short period of study at St Thomas's Hospital in London gained membership of the Royal College of Surgeons, London in 1813. He immediately joined the Army Medical Department where he rose through the ranks in a distinguished career lasting 46 years, starting as Regimental Assistant at Chelsea and then at the Royal Military Hospital in Plymouth, where he was promoted to Assistant Staff Surgeon. His postings took him to many different places, including Cape Town, South Africa, in 1817, where he served as Medical Inspector until moving to Mauritius in 1828. From there he was posted to the Island of St Helena as Inspector General of Army Hospitals. However, his meddling in the civil and military administration of the island resulted in a Court of Enquiry and his arrest. He was sent home to England and demoted to Staff Surgeon. In 1838 he became Principal Medical Officer in Trinidad and Tobago but in 1845 was again sent home, this time because of an attack of yellow fever which nearly killed him and from which he took a year to recover.

Barry was posted to Malta in 1846, to Corfu in 1851, and finally

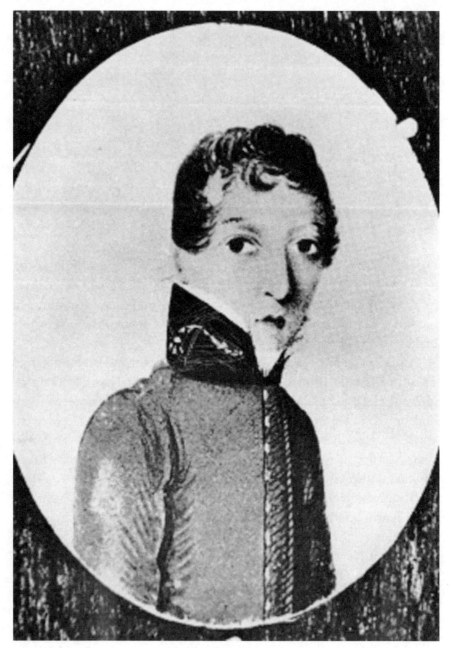

Portrait of James Barry.

ended up in Canada where he was Inspector General of Hospitals from 1857 until he retired in 1864. He then headed home to London where he died, probably of dysentery or cholera, just a year later. He was given a full military funeral and buried in Kensal Green Cemetery.

By all accounts Barry had been a difficult character throughout his career. His obituary in the *Malta Times* described him as:

> Clever and agreeable, save for the drawback of a most quarrel-some temper, and an inordinate addiction to argument, which perpetually brought the former peculiarity into play... excessively plain, of feeble proportions, and laboured under the imperfection of a ludicrously squeaking voice.[1]

Barry's voice was the focus of persistent teasing by fellow officers, whom he challenged to a duel on more than one occasion, killing one of the offenders with a shot through the lung. After that his colleagues were presumably more restrained in their teasing.

His contrary behaviour led to several reprimands for insubordination and rudeness. Shortly after his arrival in Malta, he attended the Collegiate Church of St Paul and sat in the area reserved for the clergy. His Commanding Officer, Lieutenant General Sir P Stuart, issued a garrison order describing his behaviour as 'more than disrespectful'.[2]

Despite his eccentricities, Barry was kind and generous to his patients as well as to the poor and needy. Always concerned for the welfare of the troops, he made significant improvements to their living, sanitary and dietary conditions, and coped so well with a severe cholera outbreak in Malta that he was thanked personally by the Duke of Wellington.

A fast, decisive and skilled surgeon, while in the Cape Barry carried out one of the first successful Caesarean sections; the mother named her baby son James Barry Munnik in his honour.

Only after his death in 1865 did rumours about the doctor's gender begin to circulate. Sophia Bishop, the maid at his lodgings, laid out his body but waited until after the funeral to drop the bombshell – Dr Barry was a woman. Some army colleagues said that they had suspected as much all along, others suggested that Barry was perhaps a hermaphrodite. More recently it has been speculated that he may have had androgen insensitivity syndrome, a congenital condition in which people who have male chromosomes lack the male hormone receptor and therefore do not develop secondary sexual characteristics on reaching puberty. As rumours escalated, the British Army locked Barry's records away and it was not until the 1950s that historian Isobel Rae persuaded the army to reopen the case.[3] But although this provided details of the doctor's army career, Barry's early life might have remained shrouded in mystery had it not been for the clever detective-work of Michael du Preez, a retired doctor from Cape Town.[4]

Barry arrived in Edinburgh to commence his medical studies with his so-called aunt, Mary Ann Bulkley. No records of his earlier life at the University existed, but du Preez made the connection between James Barry the doctor and another James Barry, an Irish artist whose quarrelsome temperament got him expelled from the Royal Academy. Du Preez uncovered a clear trail of documentary evidence linking the two and argues convincingly that Dr James Barry started life as Margaret Ann Bulkley, daughter of the artist's sister Mary Ann.

Margaret Ann Bulkley was born in Cork in 1789. Her father, Jeremiah Bulkley, was in the grocery trade. By the early 1800s the family had fallen on hard times and Jeremiah was detained in a debtors' prison in Dublin. Mary Ann and her daughter turned for help to Uncle James. They moved to London, where Barry, along with his radical friends, including General Francisco de Miranda, a Venezuelan revolutionary, and Dr Edward Fryer, an academic physician, supervised Margaret's education. She was probably being educated to become a governess or teacher, but after Barry's death a new plan was hatched – that she would study Medicine. Then, disguised as a man, she would accompany General de Miranda to Venezuela to practice as a (female) doctor.

In November 1809 Mary Ann Bulkley and her daughter disappeared from London, boarding the passenger ferry from Wapping to Leith with Margaret already disguised as James Barry, ostensibly Mary Ann's nephew, to begin a new life in Edinburgh. Margaret/James carried a letter of introduction to Lord Buchan, an influential friend of her late uncle, who was probably instrumental in facilitating her passage through her medical studies and her career in the army. Despite lying about her true age in order to explain her boyish features, all went well at the University and she graduated in 1812. Her thesis, dedicated to General de Miranda, must have been completed at about the time the general made an unsuccessful attempt to liberate Spanish America and was imprisoned in Cadiz, where he died of typhus in 1816. His death extinguished Barry's dream of practising medicine in Venezuela and the young doctor immediately joined the army. Why she decided on this astonishing and possibly even dangerous career and how she managed to conceal her true sex at the physical examination, we shall probably never know, but it is likely that the well-connected Lord Buchan came to her assistance.

By any standard Barry had a remarkably successful career and avoided detection for over 40 years. However there were some near misses, one in Cape Town in 1817 when she visited the Count of Las Cases with a fellow captain. The Count wrote in his journal (published in 1823):

> I mistook the captain's medical friend for his son, or nephew. The grave Doctor, who was presented to me, was a boy of 18, with a form, the manners, and the voice of a woman. But Mr Barry (such was his name) was described to be an absolute phenomenon. I was informed that he had obtained his diploma at the age of 13, after the most rigid examination, and that he had performed extraordinary cures at the Cape.[5]

Women's Struggle to Study Medicine

It was just a few years before Barry's death that another woman applied to matriculate for the MD course at the University of Edinburgh. She was refused – an action which heralded the long and bitter struggle for women's admission to Medical School, with much of the drama being played out in Edinburgh. Perhaps if the story of Margaret Bulkley, alias James Barry, had been known it could have prevented some of the conflict and eased the passage of the early pioneers.

In England as early as the 13th century there were concerns over the danger of allowing 'ignorant and unskilled persons' to practise medicine and surgery,[6] and over the years several Acts of Parliament were passed in an attempt to protect the public from the practices of quacks and charlatans. This culminated with the Medical Act of 1858, which ruled that would-be practitioners in Britain had to be registered before they could set up their plate, with registration requiring a qualification from one of 19 named examining bodies, including recognised universities and colleges. Registration in itself did not exclude women, but none of the named institutions accepted them among their students or apprentices. Until the mid-19th century they were probably rarely, if ever, asked to do so.

In the Victorian era most middle-class women were restricted to the traditional roles of wife and mother. Those without financial support had few options for earning a living, beyond working as teachers or governesses. The contention was that women were intellectually inferior to men and too frail to withstand the rigours of higher education and work outside the home. (Given the burden of toil that working-class women usually shouldered, the inference is that the term 'women', as used thus in this intensely class-stratified society, was not an inclusive term across all classes.) Regarding medicine, there were additional 'fears' about degrading women's purity. Queen Victoria herself threatened to withdraw her patronage from a medical conference if women were admitted.[7]

In the late 1850s a counter-attack began on these constraints, but for the small group of women eager to enter the profession of Medicine, gaining access to recognised college or university courses and examinations in order to qualify for registration seemed to be an insurmountable hurdle.

Interestingly, at the same time as women were struggling to be accepted into Medicine, Florence Nightingale and her team of nurses were ministering to the wounded in the war-torn Crimea. Encouraged by doctors, she later set up a nursing school in London that transformed nursing into a respectable vocation for ladies. Since no arguments regarding the frailty of women and the protection of their modesty outlawed these 'ministering angels', it seems clear that opposition to women medical graduates was, at least in part, due to the threat they might pose at a time when there was severe competition for patients. If female patients preferred female doctors, male doctors stood to lose income.

The first British woman to qualify in Medicine was Elizabeth Blackwell, whose family emigrated from Bristol to the USA, where she undertook her training. After being refused entry to 29 medical schools, she gained a place at the University of Geneva, New York, and graduated in 1849. She established the New York Infirmary for Women, then in 1858 returned to Britain where, as a holder of a foreign degree, she was able to join the medical register. Her lectures on women in medicine inspired Elizabeth Garrett (later Elizabeth Garrett-Anderson) to study Medicine. After being refused admission to all English medical schools, Garrett travelled to Scotland to try her luck at the universities of St Andrews and Edinburgh. The result was the same: in Edinburgh the poll at the physicians' meeting at which her application was discussed went against her by 18 votes to 16, and at St Andrews too she was refused admission. In the end she took private tuition from teachers at St Andrews and in 1865 she passed the London Society of Apothecaries examination, which qualified her to practise as a doctor. This route was immediately closed by the Society of Apothecaries, which changed its charter to allow only those who had studied at a recognised medical school to take their exams. However, universities in Zurich, Paris, Berne and Geneva opened their doors to women students, from 1864 onwards and Garrett travelled to the Sorbonne to gain an MD and then practised in London at St Mary's Dispensary for Women and Children. For 12 years she and Blackwell were the only two women on the medical register and able to practise in the UK.

The next onslaught on the male bastion was played out in Edinburgh in 1869 when the pioneering Sophia Jex-Blake and four other women matriculated in the Medical Faculty. Jex-Blake was born in Sussex into a middle-class family. Her father was a solicitor. The youngest of three, she showed early signs of intelligence and determination, and swiftly became bored with the elementary lessons taught at the boarding schools she attended. Her boisterous behaviour at home so upset her rather delicate mother that she was sometimes left at school during the holidays, but her parents, although somewhat startled by their daughter's behaviour, were supportive of her ambitions. When she left school in 1857 determined to continue her education, she persuaded them to allow her to attend Queen's College in London, where ladies were taught to advanced secondary school level. At last she was happy and fully occupied; she made friends with like-minded, pioneering women, one of whom was Garrett.

In 1862 Jex-Blake decided to continue her studies in Edinburgh, where she had heard that classes for women were available, particularly in Mathematics, at which she excelled. The standard of the Edinburgh classes disappointed her, but she came armed with letters of introduction to influential people and through them she met others who could give her private tuition in Maths, German and English. In May that same year Garrett arrived in Edinburgh with the hope of matriculating in Medicine at the University. With the help of Jex-Blake she spent two weeks canvassing support among the professors and although in the end the vote went against Garrett, Jex-Blake did not see this decision as irrevocable.

After six months in Edinburgh Jex-Blake left to teach English in schools in Europe before heading to the USA to visit schools for young women with a view to setting up her own establishment on her return. In Boston she met Lucy Sewall, a graduate from the newly-established New England Female Medical College who was working in the New England Hospital for Women and Children. Jex-Blake stayed with her at the hospital and inevitably was drawn into hospital life. It was at this point that she had a change of heart about her career and abandoned the idea of teaching in favour of becoming a doctor.

She wrote to the President and Fellows of Harvard University on three occasions, requesting entrance to the Medical School but was turned down each time on the pretext that: 'in our school no provision for that purpose [the education of women] has been made, or is at present contemplated'.[8] With this decision she reluctantly left Boston for New York and became one of the first students at a college attached to the New York Infirmary for Women, which opened in 1868. Jex-

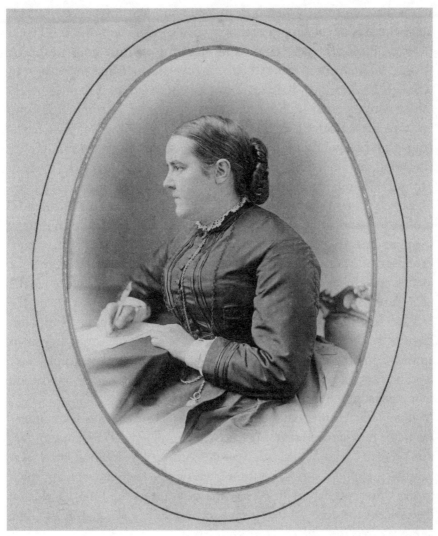

Sophia Jex-Blake.

Blake was delighted with the teaching, but after a week she received news that her father was gravely ill and hurried home, only to find that he had died. She gave up her plans to study Medicine in the USA in order to stay with her grieving family. But it was not long before she set her sights on Edinburgh 'to which so much credit is always given for its enlightened views respecting education, and where the Universities boast of their freedom from ecclesiastical and other trammels'.[9]

On her return to Edinburgh in 1869 she was introduced to two men who were avid supporters of women's further education – David Masson, Professor of Rhetoric and English Literature and Alexander Russel, the influential editor of the *Scotsman*. Her first move was to write to Professor JJ Balfour, Dean of the Medical Faculty, merely asking permission to attend medical lectures during the summer session. She then busied herself seeking support among members of the Faculty who would be voting on her request. The topic of women's university education, let alone their right to study Medicine, divided the medical professors. Sir James Young Simpson, who had previously employed Blackwell's sister Emily as his assistant, was whole-heartedly on her side. Professor James Syme was only supportive if women agreed to restrict their practice to obstetrics and gynaecology, and Robert Christison, Professor of Materia Medica and Therapeutics, asserted that the poor intellectual ability and stamina of women would lower standards in the profession. Surprisingly, the votes of both the Medical Faculty and the Senatus went in Jex-Blake's favour and she became famous overnight. But this was by no means the end of the line and her struggle was to continue for the next four years. Only someone with extraordinary fortitude and determination could have withstood the bitter opposition that met each of her requests.

It was universally assumed that subjects like Anatomy and Surgery would be taught in separate classes to male and female students, and on this pretext Claud Muirhead, Senior Assistant Physician at the Royal Infirmary, supported by a petition from nearly 200 students, appealed to the University Court to review the decision of the Senatus. Within three weeks the decision had been overturned. Jex-Blake, now at home in Sussex, received the unhappy news:

The Court, considering the difficulties at present in the way of carrying out the resolution of the Senatus, as a temporary arrangement in the interest of one lady, and not being prepared to adjudicate finally on the question whether women should be educated in the medical classes of the University, sustains the appeals and recalls the resolution of the Senatus.[10]

Masson, who represented Jex-Blake at the court meeting, thought that since the main objection to her request was that it was not worth the expense of setting up special classes for one woman, court approval might still be obtained if several women applied to study medicine at once. Russel publicised the controversy in his newspaper, and soon she had the names of four women keen to join her in the fight: 43-year-old mother of four, Isabel Thorne, who was encouraged to apply by her businessman husband; Edith Pechey and Matilda Chaplin, who had both worked with Garrett; and Helen Evans, widow of an army officer. They were later joined by two more students, Mary Anderson and Emily Bovell, forming what became known as 'the Edinburgh Seven'.

The new application, this time for matriculation to the full medical course, was considered by the Medical Faculty, Senatus and University Court, and although it faced great opposition, in the end it won their approval. This was a breakthrough of huge significance, but no time could be spared on celebrations. The matriculation exams were just a few weeks away, with compulsory papers in English, Latin and Mathematics, and a choice of two more subjects from Greek, French, Higher Maths, Natural Philosophy, Logic and Moral Philosophy. Jex-Blake found accommodation at 15 Buccleuch Place and Pechey moved in with her. Jex-Blake studied hard at the same time as coaching the others and their lodgings became a social centre and headquarters in the battles to come.

All five women who had initially enrolled passed their matriculation, with four of them among the top seven. They signed the matriculation roll in November 1869. This was a historic moment – Edinburgh became the first university in the UK to accept female undergraduates. The University regulations were changed to accommodate the women, who had to pay higher fees for the separate classes that were imposed on them but would otherwise be treated exactly as the male students. Then a snag arose. University teachers were *permitted* but not *required* to give lectures to women and since this arrangement meant extra work, not all were willing or able to oblige. It was left up to the women to arrange their lectures, Jex-Blake, as always, taking the lead. For the first winter term the lecturers in both Physiology and Chemistry agreed to teach women's classes and all went well until the exams in March 1870. The women all passed, with four of them achieving honours in both subjects. Pechey was first among those candidates taking the Chemistry exam for the first time and was therefore eligible for a Hope Scholarship. However, her success upset many of the male students. Alex Crum Brown, the Professor of Chemistry, fearing hostility, awarded the scholarships to male students ranked below her, saying that she was ineligible because she had been taught in special separate classes. He stated that he would issue the ladies with a credit for attending the ladies' class (as opposed to a standard certificate of attendance at his Chemistry lectures), although he admitted that the lectures were identical. This credit did not meet the Faculty's requirements for the medical degreee. The women appealed to the Senatus over the injustice and the vote went in their favour by a majority of one, so they were finally granted standard certificates for Chemistry. They also appealed over the subject of Pechey's Hope Scholarship, but Christison moved that:

> the authorities of the University have not passed any Resolution extending to females the right to competing for those University Prizes which have hitherto been competed for by, and were originally destined for, male students of the University...[11]

This was also carried with a majority of one and so Pechey lost her chance of a scholarship. However the publicity that followed earned the women widespread respect and support. *The Times* reported:

> [Miss Pechey] has done her sex a service, not only by vindicating their intellectual ability in an open competition with men, but still more by the temper and courtesy with which she meets her disappointment.[12]

Jex-Blake, always one for looking forward rather than back, put this disappointment behind her and set about arranging the women's lectures for the next term, but in the wake of such public controversy, several staff now found themselves too busy to help, including William Turner, Professor of Anatomy (and later Principal of the University). Masson, seconded by the Dean of Medicine, proposed to the University Council that the women should be taught in the same classes as the men. The proposal was defeated, with Professor Laycock, Professor of Practice of Medicine and Clinical Medicine, implying that some women seeking medical training could be 'basely inclined' – meaning that they were intent on becoming abortionists – and Christison suggesting that the presence of women students would increase the 'irregular behaviour' of the men.[13] Jex-Blake was forced to apply to the extra-mural schools for some of the women's teaching for the summer term. This worked well, with the women even attending the men's Natural History lectures given by Dr Alleyne Nicholson. But the following winter term (1870–71) was not so easy; Anatomy and Surgery were the subjects on the curriculum and the University teachers again refused to teach the women. Willing extra-mural teachers at Surgeon's Hall taught the women anatomical dissection and surgery in their ordinary classes. All seemed calm, but the opposition was gathering strength and with the sudden death of James Syme and the appointment of Joseph Lister to the Chair of Surgery, the tide turned. The women urgently needed access to patients in the Royal Infirmary of Edinburgh for their clinical teaching, but when Jex-Blake applied for permission it was refused. A petition signed by 500 students swung the vote in their favour, but the attitude of some male students towards their female classmates did not make things easy. In Jex-Blake's words:

> A certain proportion of the students with whom we worked became markedly offensive and insolent, and took every opportunity of practising the petty annoyances that occur to thoroughly ill-bred lads, – such as shutting doors in our faces, ostentatiously crowding into the seats we usually occupied, bursting into horse-laughs and howls when we approached, – as if a conspiracy had been formed to make our position as uncomfortable as might be.[14]

The women's allies were sure that Christison and his like-minded colleagues were behind this offensive behaviour, which reached a peak on 18 November with the Surgeons' Hall riot. An anatomy exam was scheduled and a mob of several hundred, including a group of drunk and rowdy students, was already waiting in Nicholson Street when the seven women arrived at Surgeons' Hall. As they struggled through the crowd they were heckled, jostled and pelted with mud and dirt. On reaching the building they were barred entry until a supporter opened the door and hastily ushered them inside. The exam, presided over by Dr Handyman, was interrupted when the rioters shoved a live sheep into the room. The publicity surrounding the day's events won the women public goodwill but it turned the University against them.

On 2 January 1871 the annual public meeting was held to appoint the Royal Infirmary's board of managers and since the issue of admitting women students to the wards would certainly come up for debate, both Jex-Blake and her opponents were keen to be represented. After the Surgeons' Hall riot publicity, the meeting proved so popular that it had to be moved across the street from the Edinburgh Council Chamber to St Giles Cathedral. Jex-Blake spoke at the meeting, claiming:

> This I do know, that the riot was not wholly or mainly due to the students at Surgeons' Hall. I know that Dr Christison's class assistant was one of the leading rioters, and the foul language he used could only be excused on the supposition I heard that he was intoxicated. I do not say that Dr Christison knew of or sanctioned his presence, but I do say that I think he would not have been there, had he thought the doctor would have strongly objected to his presence.[15]

An immediate appeal from Christison obliged Jex-Blake to withdraw the word 'intoxicated', but she added: 'If Dr Christison prefers that I should say he used the language when sober, I will withdraw the other supposition.'[16]

The retiring members of the board were re-elected for another year, effectively blocking the women access to the wards for that period. At another public meeting held two weeks later to consider the plight of the Edinburgh seven, a petition expressing the hope that the managers would allow them access to hospital facilities was presented, signed by nearly 1,000 Edinburgh women. A Mrs Nichol, who said she spoke for a further 1,300 women, observed:

> If the students studying at present in the Infirmary cannot contemplate with equanimity the presence of ladies as fellow students, how is it possible that they can possess either the scientific spirit, or the personal purity of mind, which alone would justify their presence in the female wards during the most delicate operation on, and examination of, female patients?[17]

But still nothing changed. Furthermore, as a result of her impulsive speech in the cathedral, Jex-Blake received a defamation writ from Christison's assistant, Mr Craig, seeking compensation of £1,000 for accusing him of leading the Surgeons' Hall riot. The campaign had now become personal and Christison was hoping she would be discredited when the case came to court in May 1871. The public seating was packed when the jury announced its verdict; it found in favour of Craig, but awarded him damages of only a farthing. However, this was not quite the end of the affair: the court later decided that Jex-Blake should pay the full costs of the hearing – £916.

At the University all the women had passed their exams in March 1871, but a new problem arose. According to regulations, candidates for medical degrees were allowed to take extra-mural classes in only four subjects; but as Jex-Blake pointed out to the Senatus, having received extra-mural tuition in four subjects, the women had nowhere else to turn as the University lecturers refused to teach them. She suggested either appointing more lecturers to teach the women, at the women's expense, or allowing them to take more than four extra-mural classes. Having sought legal advice, Senatus was adamant:

> We are satisfied that the University has all along been and must still be regarded as an institution devoted exclusively to the education of male students. The result of this view, in our opinion,

is that males alone have any right to demand, and on complying with the regulations of the University to obtain, admission to the privilege of Studentship.[18]

Fearing that the University would exclude them from their first professional examination, which the five original women students were now ready to take, they sought advice from the Lord Advocate. His decision was that, having allowed the five to matriculate, and at the time having changed the rules to state that they had 'the same rights and privileges as those enjoyed by male students',[19] the University could not exclude them from taking professional exams. Four of the women immediately took and passed the exam but Jex-Blake, who had been organising courses for three new women students, decided to delay until she was better prepared. Now at the end of their second year of study, the group needed assurance that they could complete the course. At a University Council meeting, Dr Alexander Wood, armed with a petition bearing the signatures of 9,000 supporters, moved that the University was honour-bound to allow the women to complete their degree courses. Christison and his ally, Turner, were ready with a counter-attack and the motion was defeated by 107 votes to 97.

A short period of elation came in 1872 with the election of a board of managers for Edinburgh Royal Infirmary that was supportive of the women; Masson moved that all students regardless of their sex should be admitted to the wards, all the opponents walked out, and the motion was carried. The excitement at this victory was intense, but two weeks later some board members claimed that the vote had been unconstitutional as representatives of Scottish firms were allowed to vote and the matter was referred to the courts, with the case not due to be heard for six months. With Scotland's Lord Advocate on her side, Jex-Blake believed that she would win the case, which was heard in July. She was right. The Lord Ordinary, Lord Gifford, ruled in the women's favour, stating that:

According to the existing constitution and regulations of the said University of Edinburgh, the pursuers are entitled to be

admitted to the study of medicine in the said University, and...
on completing the prescribed studies... are entitled to proceed to
examination for degrees in manner prescribed by the regulations
of the University of Edinburgh.[20]

This truly great victory was achieved at the expense of Jex-Blake's
own career. Preparing for the court case, writing articles for the press
and delivering lectures meant that she had neglected her studies. She
had five weeks left to prepare for her first professional examination
in October when the University appealed against Lord Gifford's
decision and her studies were again interrupted. She failed in all three
subjects (Natural History, Botany and Chemistry). This was not only
a setback for her professionally but also highly embarrassing, as it
was fuel to those opponents of women's education who thought
them intellectually inferior to men. Jex-Blake argued publicly that the
marking of her papers had been biased, but others were unconvinced.
However, her fighting spirit soon rallied and she set to work gaining
support for the women's cause. In December 1872 the voting of firms
for the board of managers of the Royal Infirmary was finally declared
valid and the pro-women board came into office just two weeks before
their term ended. Fortunately this was time enough to approve the
admittance of women students to the hospital wards. Although they
were to be taught separately from the men and restricted to just a few
wards, supportive senior staff, namely physician Dr George Balfour
and surgeon Dr Heron Watson, set aside time to teach them, the latter
on Sunday mornings, which his opponents denounced as an offence
against Sabbath observance. However the Lord Provost, James Cowan,
silenced them by attending one of the classes himself and declaring it to
be 'a truly Sabbatical work of healing'.[21]

Despite the victory at the Royal Infirmary the women were still
unsure of their chances of qualifying at the University and were
already exploring other possibilities when the appeal hearing of the
Lord Ordinary's decision took place. A panel of judges overturned his
decision by a majority of seven to five, thereby not allowing the women
to qualify, and ordered them to pay £850 costs.

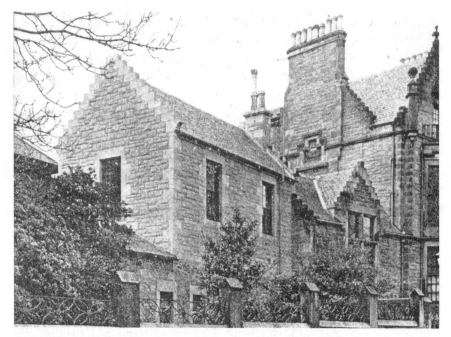

Edinburgh Hospital and Dispensary for Women, later Bruntsfield Hospital.

Since they could not take their medical degree exams, this was the end of the road for the Edinburgh Seven. The University, having been the first to admit women students, rejected them just four years later. But it was not the end for their careers. Their battle moved to London, where it became a political fight for equal educational rights for women.

Jex-Blake's immense energy was now focused on the political campaign to change the law, but she was also instrumental in establishing the UK's first women's medical school, the London School of Medicine for Women, which opened in 1874 and later amalgamated with the Royal Free Hospital to become the Royal Free Hospital Medical School. Twelve of the first 14 students had previously studied in Edinburgh and were now keen to complete their training. But despite the efforts of a group of supportive MPs to amend the Medical Act of 1858 to include women, the students were still unable to sign the Medical Register in Britain unless a recognised body allowed them to sit their examinations. A chink of light appeared when the General Medical Council, the body in charge of the medical register, debated the issue and came up with an ambiguous statement including the following: 'The Council are not prepared to say that women ought to be excluded from the profession',[22] and in 1876, after several abortive attempts to change the law, MP Russell Gurney's Enabling Bill, which gave all medical examining bodies the right to admit women, was finally passed at Westminster. The College of Physicians in Dublin was the first examining body willing to open its doors to women, and Jex-Blake and Pechey, having first spent two months in Berne, Switzerland, to obtain an MD degree, passed the Irish exams in 1877 and their names were finally added to the medical register.

The tide of opinion was clearly turning in favour of higher education for women. In 1877 the senate of London University voted in favour of admitting female medical students – the first, and for 10 years the only British university to allow women to graduate.

Between 1874 and 1877 Jex-Blake had been busy with the administrative task of running the London School of Medicine for Women, but when she returned from Dublin with her medical degree after an absence of several months she found that her chance of gaining the role of Honorary School Secretary, which she had assumed would be hers, was under threat.

In her absence the executive council had decided that with her outspoken and confrontational style, she was not the right person to lead the school. Eventually, to avoid open conflict and at the expense of her own medical career, Isabel Thorne agreed to take the post. Following this disappointment Jex-Blake returned to Edinburgh, where she set up in practice in 1878 as the first female doctor in the city. She later opened the Edinburgh Hospital and Dispensary for Women.

In 1886 the Royal Colleges of Physicians and Surgeons in both Glasgow and Edinburgh established a joint exam in Medicine and Surgery open to men and women, but Scottish women still had problems finding medical classes to attend. Jex-Blake was called upon to help them and eventually she was convinced that an Edinburgh School of Medicine for Women was the answer. This establishment opened in Surgeons' Square in 1887 with eight students. Jex-Blake was Director and Dean and several of her old supporters, including Balfour and

Watson, were on the executive committee. Jex-Blake found clinical training for the students at Leith Hospital and the school flourished for a few years, but her authoritarian style led to its downfall. Two students, sisters Ina and Grace Cadell, who were outspoken in their opposition to what they saw as Jex-Blake's over-domineering ways, were eventually expelled. Joined by another student, Elsie Inglis, they set up the Medical College for Women in Chambers Street in 1889, in direct competition with Jex-Blake's school and with lower fees. At first their students travelled to Glasgow Royal Infirmary for clinical teaching, but in 1892 they gained access to the wards at the Royal Infirmary of Edinburgh. From this point Jex-Blake's school could not compete and it closed in 1898 after 12 years, having trained 28 doctors, with a total of 70 students attending some courses.

Jex-Blake's work at the hugely successful Edinburgh Hospital and Dispensary for Women, which later became the Bruntsfield Hospital, continued until 1899 when she retired to a farm in Sussex. She died there in 1912.

The other six members of the Edinburgh Seven all retained an active interest in the struggle and four qualified and practised medicine. Edith Pechey studied at the London Medical School for Women and in 1877, along with Jex-Blake, she obtained an MD in Berne and passed the medical examinations in Dublin. She practised in Leeds before heading for Bombay where she ran the Cama Hospital for Women and Children. She was later appointed to the senate of the University of Bombay. Isabel Thorne became a student at the London School of Medicine for Women, of which she was a council member, in 1874. Because of family commitments she could not go with her contemporaries to Berne to obtain an MD and so could not sit the exams with them in Dublin. In 1877 she gave up her aspirations to become a doctor to take the role of honorary secretary to the London School of Medicine for Women, a post which she held until 1906. Emily Bovell gained an MD in Paris in 1877 and sat the Irish College exams for medical registration. She worked in the New Hospital for Women in London from 1878 to 1881 and she then moved to Nice because she was suffering from TB.

However, in a single year, 1871, Helen Evans, Matilda Chaplin and Mary Anderson gave up their medical studies for marriage. Evans married Alexander Russel, with whom she had three children; after her husband's sudden death of a heart attack in 1876, she became a member of the executive committee of the Edinburgh School of Medicine for Women. Chaplin married William Ayrton, Professor of Physics at the University of Edinburgh. They moved to Tokyo, where she founded a school of Midwifery. On their return to London she studied at the London School of Medicine for Women, obtained an MD from Paris in 1879 and sat her final exams at the College of Physicians in Dublin before setting up in private practice. Anderson, sister of Garrett-Anderson's husband, married a Mr Marshall, but when he died a few months later she joined the London School of Medicine for Women to complete her studies. She gained an MD in Paris in 1879 and passed the Irish exams to obtain her medical registration. She then worked in the New Hospital for Women in London until 1895 when she moved to Cannes due to ill health.

The University of Edinburgh finally allowed female medical students to graduate in 1894 and the first female doctors graduated in 1896. Even then they were not permitted to attend all the medical classes but had to find their own tuition, just as Jex-Blake and her pioneering colleagues had done.

Among the earliest female medical graduates was Elsie Inglis, who had previously trained at the Medical College for Women, receiving clinical teaching at Glasgow Royal Infirmary. In 1892 she took the exams of the Royal Colleges of Physicians and Surgeons of Edinburgh and the Faculty of Physicians and Surgeons of Glasgow, which she passed with high marks, and became a registered practitioner. She set up practice in Edinburgh and in 1899 she also graduated in Medicine from the University of Edinburgh. She opened a small hospital at 11 George Square for poor women and children; it moved to larger premises in the High Street in 1904. This was called 'The Hospice' and comprised surgical, gynaecological and accident departments as well as a dispensary.

Inglis soon became well known in Edinburgh for her medical skill, her energy and her kindness to her patients and their families. In 1905 she accepted a consultant post at the Bruntsfield Hospital, an appointment which had been blocked by Jex-Blake in 1899 because of their past disagreements. On this occasion the hospital managers insisted, causing Jex-Blake to sever her connections with the hospital. In 1907 Inglis was appointed senior consultant at the hospital, which later amalgamated with The Hospice. During these pre-war years Inglis was very involved with the women's suffrage movement. Although never a militant, she was honorary secretary of the Edinburgh National Society for Women's Suffrage and often addressed public meetings.

When war broke out in 1914 Inglis was determined to use her medical skills in the war effort and was surprised and disappointed when the Royal Army Medical Corp (RAMC) representative at Edinburgh Castle responded with: 'My good lady, go home and sit still'.[23] Despite the acute need for doctors, the unwavering attitude of the War Office was to ban women from the war zone. Inglis took things into her own hands, persuading the Scottish and National Women's Suffrage Societies to fund and organise field hospitals run entirely by women, and offer these units to Allied governments.

This highly successful initiative, which evolved into the Scottish Women's Hospitals, was both inspired and led by Inglis. Belgium, France and Serbia were the first to take up the offer of units and she was instrumental in setting up the first unit in the medieval abbey of Royaumont near Paris. She then travelled to Serbia, which was facing the threat of invasion from Austria-Hungary. She arrived in the middle of a typhus epidemic and along with the friendly Colonel William Hunter from the RAMC she sorted out the quarantine and disinfection requirements needed to prevent spread of the infection via body lice. Hunter later said of her:

> I have never met with anyone who gave me so deep an impression of single-mindedness, gentle-heartedness, clear and purposeful vision, wise judgement, and absolutely fearless disposition.[24]

Inglis and her team remained in Serbia as the German army advanced, staying behind when Serbia was lost to the Allies and others had opted to retreat. Those remaining were taken prisoner by the Germans and

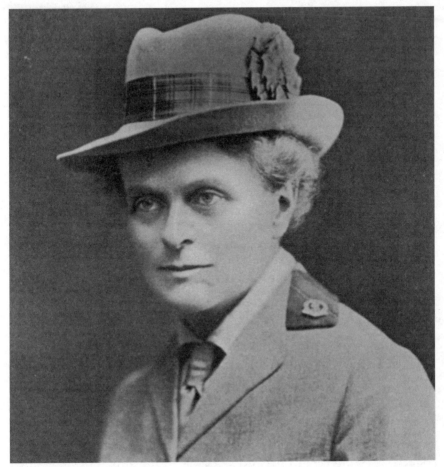

Elsie Inglis.

worked at the Czar Lazar Barrack prisoner-of-war hospital, where, in appalling conditions, they treated a never-ending stream of the wounded while suffering from severe cold and food shortages throughout the winter of 1915. In early 1916 they were repatriated. On their arrival home on 29 February they were dubbed 'The Scottish Heroines'. The press described Inglis, then aged 52, as:

> A bright-faced little woman in a grey uniform who spoke modestly, almost shyly, of her work among the Serbians and referred to the risks she had run as if they were everyday and commonplace.[25]

In April she was awarded the Order of the White Eagle for war service by the Crown Prince of Serbia, then in August she was off again, this time on a ship heading for Archangel in Russia, leading a unit requested by the Serbian government to provide a hospital for two Serbian divisions fighting with the Russians. From Archangel they travelled by train to Odessa, a journey of nine days, and then on to Medjidia in Romania, where they set up their hospital in a barrack and were soon treating thousands of wounded soldiers. But three weeks later, as the Germans advanced, they were ordered to evacuate to Galatz, a large Romanian port on the Danube. When they were halted at Braila, where the river was blocked, Inglis set up the unit with operating theatre and wards and again treated thousands of wounded soldiers. When Braila was threatened by German invasion the team moved the unit to Galatz, and in early January 1917 this too was evacuated, with Inglis and four others remaining with the patients till the last minute and only by luck finding a boat to take them to Reni in the Ukraine.

Inglis and the unit spent eight months in Reni, mostly treating Russians rather than Serbs. With the Russians involved in their revolution from March onwards and their army in disarray, the situation became chaotic. Inglis was still keen to help the Serbian divisions and in August the unit moved to join the Serbs in Bressarabia (then part of Romania, now part of Moldova) where the hospital was housed under canvas. It was here that Inglis, who had secretly known since before the war that she was suffering from cancer, became seriously ill, but she assured everyone that she would recover. Inglis was only interested in gaining safe passage for the Serbs and once this was assured she agreed to go home, but by the time the unit left for Archangel at the end of October 1917 she was virtually bed-ridden. They boarded ship on 9 November and with an ice-breaker clearing their path, the convoy sailed for Newcastle. Arriving there on 24 November, Inglis, extremely weak and in great pain, got up to bid farewell to the Serbs on board. She collapsed and was taken to the nearby Station Hotel where she died the next day. Her obituary in *The Lancet* said: 'Elsie Inglis gave her life for her country and its allies as truly as any soldier in the trenches has ever done and as cheerfully.'[26]

CHAPTER 5

Four Men Famous Beyond Medicine

THESE DAYS, RIGID UK government quotas regulate the number of students enrolled to study Medicine each year. Competition is fierce and places are highly prized, with most medical students at the University of Edinburgh staying the course and qualifying as doctors. Course content is regulated and more or less confined to topics directly related to the practice of medicine, but things were very different in earlier times.

In the 18th and early 19th centuries education was far less formalised and it was quite common for students as young as 14 to matriculate at the University. The Medical curriculum was broad, with courses in Chemistry, Botany, and Natural Sciences – including Zoology and Geology – as well as Clinical Medicine.

Unlike most other universities in the UK and continental Europe, Edinburgh was a civic-funded university, unfettered by political and religious discrimination. Those unable to attend other universities because of their beliefs found a haven of learning at Edinburgh and it became a centre of free thinking. This era of the Scottish Enlightenment peaked in the 18th century when Edinburgh attracted intellectuals from around the globe.

Until the late 19th century scientific studies were mainly practised by the landed gentry, clergymen and a few free-thinking academics. Since the Faculty of Science at the University of Edinburgh did not exist until 1893, many of those interested in science before this time opted to study Medicine. This chapter celebrates four famous students of the Edinburgh Medical School who went on to make their names in other fields, but whose experiences during their time at the University influenced their lives. James Hutton, Joseph Black, Charles Darwin and Arthur Conan Doyle.

Hutton, often dubbed the founder of modern geology, was an energetic, imaginative and original gentleman-scientist who admirably typifies the polymath of the Scottish Enlightenment. Although he was without academic ambition and never held a university post, he was a leading light of the period, rubbing shoulders with other scholars including Adam Smith (economist and philosopher), Joseph Black (chemist), Adam Ferguson (philosopher and historian), William Robertson (historian, theologian and Principal of the University of Edinburgh 1762–93), David Hume (philosopher, economist and historian), Lord Monboddo (judge), as well as John Clerk of Eldin (artist) and his brother George Clerk Maxwell (agriculturist), and a younger group consisting of John Playfair (scientist and mathematician), John Clerk junior and Sir James Hall of Dunglass (geologist).

Hutton was born and bred in Edinburgh, the son of a merchant, and after attending the Royal High School he proceeded to the University at the age of 14 to study Law. While there he attended Chemistry lectures that stimulated his life-long passion for the subject. He practised Law for a short time, but as the life of a legal apprentice did not appeal he returned to the University in 1744 to study Medicine. Hutton went on to Paris to study Chemistry and Anatomy and then moved to Leiden where he wrote a thesis entitled *On Circulation of Blood in a Microcosm,* graduating in 1749.

While still students, Hutton and his friend James Davie invented a method for using soot to manufacture sal ammoniac, a major ingredient of smelling salts. The two friends went into partnership in 1749 and, with Davie running the production plant, grew rich on the proceeds. This relieved Hutton of having to practise Medicine, with which he was not particularly enamoured. On returning from Leiden he spent the next 14 years studying and practising agriculture at Sligh Houses, a farm in Berwickshire that he had inherited from his father. He travelled throughout Britain, France, Holland and Belgium, often on foot, to

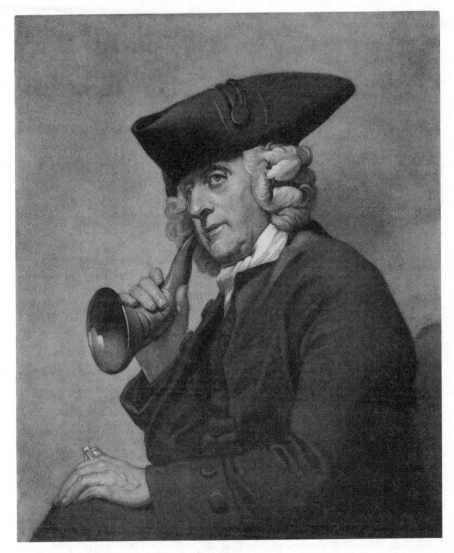

James Hutton.

learn about modern agricultural methods and over the next 40 years he wrote a book, *Elements of Agriculture*, which remained unpublished. It was on these expeditions that his lifelong fascination for geology began. In a letter to his friend and neighbour, Sir John Hall of Dunglass, he recounted how fond he had become of studying the surface of the earth, saying he was 'looking with anxious curiosity into every pit, or

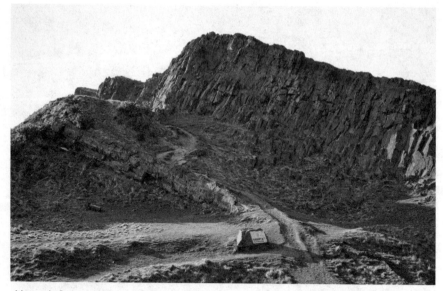

Hutton's Section of Salisbury Crags, used to prove the Plutonic theory of rock formation.

ditch, or bed of a river that fell in his way'.[1] This interest culminated in his *Theory of the Earth,* published first as a paper by the Royal Society of Edinburgh in 1788 and later as a book.

In 1767 Hutton gave up farming and returned to Edinburgh, where he lived with his three sisters in a house on St John's Hill with a fine view of Salisbury Crags. Today Hutton's Section of the Crags marks the most famous geological site in Edinburgh, showing practical proof of the Plutonic theory of rock formation.

Hutton then set about developing his theory of the Earth, travelling extensively throughout the country to observe geological formations, often accompanied by his friend John Clerk of Eldin, whose artistic talents provided accurate geological drawings of their findings. The chemist Joseph Black (another Edinburgh medical graduate) was also a lifelong friend. Black, Adam Smith and Hutton founded the Oyster Club whose select membership met weekly to discuss topical issues, often Hutton's most recent exploits and theories. But it was not until the Royal Society of Edinburgh was founded in 1783 that Hutton went public with his ideas. There he presented papers on his geological findings as well as on Chemistry, Meteorology, the Natural Sciences and the origins of speech and writing, but it is for his theories of Geology that he is rightly famed.

When Hutton was born in 1726 it was believed by the Christian world that the Earth was around 6,000 years old. This figure was deduced by Archbishop James Ussher, Primate of all Ireland between 1625 and 1656 and scholar of chronology, who pronounced that: 'Which beginning of time fell upon the entrance of the night preceding the twenty-third day of Octob. in the year 4004 [BC].'[2] This date was added to the English Bible and to question its wisdom amounted to heresy. From his observations over many years Hutton overturned this view with his theory, now called 'Deep Time'. He recognised that the rocks of the Earth's surface were, and had always been, eroded by wind and water, while at the same time others were deposited as sediments, uplifted by earthquakes and brought to the surface by volcanic eruptions, in an ongoing cycle. He concluded that the Earth's surface could have been destroyed and rebuilt an infinite number of times and, realising that rock building and destruction were slow processes taking place over an extremely long time period, he deduced that the Earth was not a few thousand but millions of years old; even speculating that it had 'no vestige of a beginning, – no prospect of an end'.[3] In his biography of Hutton, John Playfair pays tribute to his fantastic energy and his fascination with the world at large, saying that 'such a new and sublime conclusion' could only have been reached by 'a mind not fettered by prejudice, nor swayed by authority'.[4]

To support his theory Hutton found structures referred to as unconformities, famously at Siccar Point in East Lothian, where horizontal sandstone strata overlie much older, uplifted, vertical layers of schist. Playfair, who accompanying Hutton on this expedition, recalled:

On us who saw these phenomena for the first time, the impression made will not easily be forgotten… We felt ourselves necessarily carried back to the time when the schistus on which we stood was yet at the bottom of the sea, and when the sandstone before us was only beginning to be deposited, in the shape of sand or mud, from the waters of a superincumbent ocean.[5]

Hutton's second original observation was that crystalline rocks such as granite and basalt are volcanic in nature, heated underground to a molten lava that could then flow over, through and between layers of sedimentary rock. This was called the Plutonic theory (after Pluto, Roman god of the underworld) and it contradicted the more popular Neptunist theory (after Neptune, Roman god of the sea) favoured by other natural scientists at the time who believed that granite was the oldest type of rock, formed in water when conditions on the planet were 'very different from the present day'. Hutton travelled all over Scotland seeking evidence for his theory and eventually convinced himself and his companions, Clerk of Eldin and Playfair, with the sight of granite veins and dykes at Glen Tilt in Perthshire, on the Isle of Arran and Salisbury Crags in Edinburgh. These observations indicated that fluid granite had penetrated between the layers of sedimentary rock before solidifying and must therefore be the younger rock.

The conflicting Plutonic and Neptunist theories were much debated in Edinburgh society but, at the time of his death in 1797, Hutton's theories were still not universally accepted. According to Playfair this was at least partly due to the tortuous manner of Hutton's writing, which many declared unreadable:

> These defects produce a degree of obscurity astonishing to those who knew him, and who heard him every day converse with no less clearness and precision, than animation and force.[6]

Hutton's work finally gained acceptance, thanks to Playfair whose *Illustrations of the Huttonian Theory* was published five years after Hutton's death,[7] and to the famous geologist Charles Lyell, born in the year that Hutton died, who always acknowledged Hutton's major contribution to geology.

Without Hutton's demonstration that the Earth is millions of years old Charles Darwin, another Edinburgh Medical School alumnus, could not have proposed his theory of evolution by natural selection in 1859, since for this process to generate the diversity of species we see today the world must be older than a few thousand years. Just 50

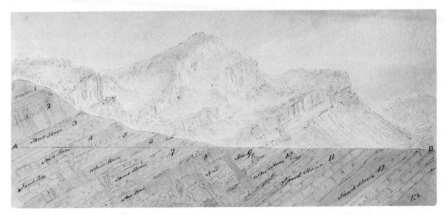

Geological drawing of Hutton's Section by John Clerk of Eldin.

years ago a rudimentary form of Darwin's theory was discovered in Hutton's *Elements of Agriculture*, a version of which, running to 2,138 pages of impenetrable prose, titled *An Investigation of the Principles of Knowledge*, was published in 1794. The book contains a chapter on selection in which Hutton expounds his theory. He noted that among dogs that relied on

> nothing but swiftness of foot, and quickness of sight [for survival] the most defective in respect of those necessary qualities, would be the most subject to perish, and that those who employed them in greatest perfection would be best preserved, consequently, would be those who would remain, to preserve themselves, and to continue the race [On the other hand if a keen sense of smell was] more necessary to the sustenance of the animal, the natural tendency of the race, acting upon the same principle of seminal variation, would be to change the qualities of the animal, and to produce a race of well scented hounds, instead of those who catch their prey by swiftness.[8]

This seems to anticipate Darwin's theory by more than 50 years but, unlike Darwin, Hutton only envisaged evolution within, and not between, species, and remained a firm believer in the Creation as described in Genesis.

Joseph Black was a contemporary of Hutton's, being just two years his senior, and therefore also enjoying the society of the unique mix of great men in Edinburgh at the time of the Enlightenment. In adult life he was a close friend of Hutton's but his childhood was very different.

Black was born in Bordeaux, France, into a family of wine merchants, one of 13 children of a Scots mother and Irish father. He was educated at home by his mother until he was 12 when he was sent to school in Belfast. At the age of 18 he went to the University of Glasgow to study Medicine. He was enthralled by the chemistry lectures given by the Professor of Medicine, William Cullen, and for three years worked as his laboratory assistant.

In 1752, after four years' study in Glasgow, Black transferred to Edinburgh where he joined his academically inclined relations on his mother's side of the family – he and his cousin, Adam Ferguson (later Professor of Moral Philosophy), both lodged with another cousin, James Russel (later Professor of Natural Philosophy). Black continued his medical studies and gained his MD in 1754. While he was a medical student Black carried out experiments on magnesia alba (magnesium carbonate) that led to his momentous discovery – of carbon dioxide, which he called 'fixed air'. Black read a paper on this to the Philosophical Society of Edinburgh in 1755 and published it in a pamphlet a year later, unleashing a revolution in chemistry. Air had been thought to be an element, but with the realisation that it was a mixture of gases, chemists soon unravelled the composition of the atmosphere, identifying another of its constituents, oxygen, which they called vital air, as essential for respiration, combustion and rusting.

Adam Ferguson later wrote in his obituary of Black for the Royal Society of Edinburgh:

Before Joseph Black offered himself a candidate for a degree in medicine, he had already made his discovery of Fixed Air; that is to say, of an elastic fluid, which being fixed in calcareous and alkaline substances, is dispelled from them in their calcinations by fire, or effervescence with acids, leaving a residuum, which, in the absence of this air with which it had been combined, becomes

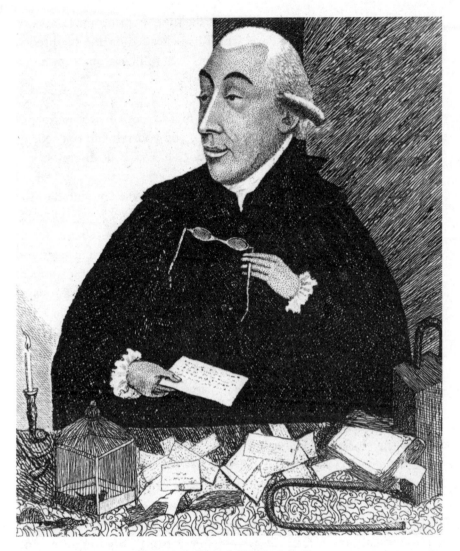

Caricature of Joseph Black by John Kay.

caustic; a quality which it retains until the air of which it was deprived is again restored...

The air obtained in this experiment has its peculiar qualities. Besides that of being fixable in stone, it is heavier than common air, its specific gravity being nearly double. Flame is extinguished, and animals are suffocated in it equally as in water.[9]

Most prominent among chemists at the time was Antoine Lavoisier, a gentleman-scientist from Paris who was beheaded during the French Revolution. He always acknowledged his debt to Black, and sent him a copy of his experiments on respiration saying:

It is but just you should be one of the first to receive information of the progress made in a career which you yourself had opened, and in which all of us here consider ourselves as your disciples.[10]

When Black's former mentor, William Cullen, was appointed to the Chair of Chemistry in Edinburgh in 1757, Black stepped into his shoes as Regius Professor of the Practice of Medicine at the University of Glasgow. It was here that he worked on his theory of latent heat and specific heat but, although he presented this work at the Philosophical and Literary Society in Glasgow and discussed it with generations of students, he never published it.

While in Glasgow Black befriended James Watt, the famous steam engine manufacturer. Watt was keen to set up an instrument-making workshop but was barred by the Glasgow Guild of Hammermen because of his lack of formal training. Black came to his rescue by offering a workshop in the University, and thereafter became Watt's mentor and friend – an interesting relationship considering the importance of latent heat to the workings of a steam engine. As Black had never published his discoveries on latent heat, Watt apparently re-discovered them in the process of trying to improve the working of the steam engine.

Black returned to Edinburgh in 1766 to succeed Cullen in the Chair of Chemistry, and from then on he concentrated on teaching and his large medical practice. By all accounts he was a highly organised and well-loved teacher, regularly attracting more than 200 students to his lectures.

Black, who never married, retired in 1797 and died in Edinburgh in 1799, aged 71. He was buried in Greyfriars churchyard. Ferguson fondly described Black as follows:

His aspect was comely, his manner unaffected and plain, and as he never had any thing about him for ostentation, he was at all times precisely what the occasion required, and nothing more... Every thing being done in its proper time and place, he ever seemed to have leisure in store...[11]

And, as Hutton was a close friend and companion of Black's, Ferguson contrasts the two characters thus: 'Black was serious, but not morose; Hutton playful, but not petulant. The one never cracked a joke, the other never uttered a sarcasm.'[12] For such an organised man, the manner of Black's death seems appropriate:

Being at table... and having the cup in his hand when the last stroke of his pulse was to be given, he appeared to have set it down on his knees, which were joined together, and in this action expired, without spilling a drop – as if an experiment had been purposely made, to evince the facility with which he departed.[13]

The University of Edinburgh's most celebrated student, Charles Darwin, attended the Medical School for only two years, but with the bicentennial celebrations of Darwin's birth in 2009 coinciding with 150 years since the publication of *On the Origin of Species*, several historians have reappraised the influence of his early studies on his later work. They contend that the seeds of Darwin's world-shattering theory were sown during his time in Edinburgh, when he was an impressionable young man.

Darwin grew up in Shropshire, the second son of Emma Wedgwood and Robert Darwin. His father, a country doctor, was himself the son of a doctor, Erasmus Darwin, author of *Zoonomia* (1794) in which it is proposed that life arose from tiny, simple life forms. It was a forerunner to the evolutionary theories proposed by the French scientist Jean-Baptiste Lamarck and by his own grandson.

Darwin was an outdoors, sports-loving child and in his memoirs he recalls being told by his father, 'You care for nothing but shooting, dogs and rat-catching, and you will be a disgrace to yourself and all your family.'[14] When he was 16, his father decided that he 'was doing

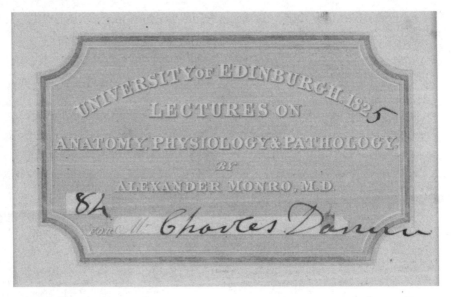

Charles Darwin's matriculation ticket for his Anatomy, Physiology and Pathology Class.

no good at school'[15] and sent him to medical school. Darwin arrived in Edinburgh in October 1825, accompanied by his elder brother, Erasmus, who had earlier begun his medical studies in Cambridge but now opted to do his external hospital study in Edinburgh. The young men were following in the footsteps of their father and grandfather, who had both studied Medicine at the University of Edinburgh.

The Darwin brothers lodged with a Mrs MacKay at 11 Lothian Street, just behind the new University buildings, now the University's Old College. Although the street has since been demolished, the site of their lodgings is marked with a plaque in South College Street. They entered a city that was humming with vitality. Arriving with notes of introduction to members of elite social circles, the brothers were soon involved in city life, and Darwin's letters home are full of stories of attending the theatre, concerts and assemblies.

During the summer before he enrolled Darwin had enjoyed attending some of his father's patients, so they both thought he would make a successful doctor. But in his autobiography, written for his family years later, he admits that, with the exception of Chemistry lectures given by Professor Thomas Hope, he found Medicine intolerably dull, recalling that, 'Dr Duncan's lectures on Materia Medica at 8 o'clock on a winter's morning are something fearful to remember.'[16] Although he regularly attended clinical teaching in the wards of the old Royal Infirmary in Infirmary Street, he found some of the cases distressing. His worst experience of all was in the operating theatre:

> I also attended on two occasions the operating theatre in the hospital at Edinburgh, and saw two very bad operations, one on a child, but I rushed away before they were completed. Nor did I ever attend again, for hardly any inducement would have been strong enough to make me do so; this being long before the blessed days of chloroform. The two cases fairly haunted me for many a long year.[17]

Clearly he was too squeamish for a career in Medicine, but after a summer of outdoor pursuits, including a trip to North Wales hillwalking with friends and riding with his sister Caroline, he returned for a second year, this time without his brother, who had gone back to Cambridge.

Fortunately the medical degree included courses in the natural sciences giving Darwin ample opportunity to pursue his interests and develop his skills in these fields. In Erasmus's absence he made new friends who shared his interests. One of these was Robert Grant, an Edinburgh medical graduate 16 years his senior who later became Professor of Comparative Anatomy and Zoology at University College, London. Grant was one of the radical intellectual Edinburgh set. He had studied Zoology in Paris and was an enthusiastic supporter of the modern theory of 'transmutation' – evolution – proposed by Lamarck. At the time he was busy searching for evidence of evolutionary links between species of marine invertebrates and published his findings regularly, often in the *Edinburgh New Philosophical Journal*. Grant scoured the tidal pools along the shores of the Firth of Forth at Leith and Newhaven for specimens and Darwin accompanied him on some of these trips. At his rented house on the shore at Prestonpans, Grant taught Darwin how to dissect, examine under the microscope and classify the specimens, while looking for minute anatomical similarities and differences which might provide evidence for evolutionary links between the species. Surely these experiences must have influenced Darwin's thinking in later life, although in his memoirs he recalls that on one of their walks:

> [Grant]... burst forth in high admiration of Lamarck and his views on evolution. I listened in silent astonishment, and as far as I can judge, without any effect on my mind. I had previously read the *Zoonomia* of my grandfather, in which similar views are maintained, but without producing any effect on me. Nevertheless it is possible that the hearing rather early in life such views maintained and praised may have favoured my upholding them under a different form in my *Origin of Species*.[18]

In Darwin's time the University of Edinburgh's Natural History Museum in Old College was one of the largest and finest in Britain. It was here that he gravitated when bored with lectures, and here that he met the founder and keeper of the museum collection, Robert Jameson, Regius Professor of Natural History. Jameson was a geologist, a convinced Lamarckian, and editor of the *Edinburgh New Philosophical Journal*. Despite Hutton's observations on volcanic rock formations in and around Edinburgh, Jameson was a Neptunist, still believing that all rocks were formed from layered deposits in an ancient ocean. Darwin evidently disagreed:

> Equally striking is the fact that I... heard Professor Jameson, in a field lecture at Salisbury Crags... with volcanic rocks all around us, and say it was a fissure filled with sediment from above, adding with a sneer that there were men who maintained that it had been injected from beneath in a molten condition. When I think of this lecture, I do not wonder that I determined never to attend to Geology.[19]

At the museum Darwin had many stimulating discussions with the curator, Mr Macgillivray, later Professor of Natural History at the

University of Aberdeen, and was taught taxidermy by John Edmonstone, a former slave from Georgetown, Guyana, who had arrived in Glasgow with his owner in 1817. Edmonstone had accompanied the eccentric British naturalist Charles Waterton on his travels in Guyana and South America and now earned a living as a taxidermist, a skill Waterton had taught him. Darwin paid him just one guinea for 40 lessons, declaring that he

> gained his livelihood by stuffing birds, which he did excellently; he gave me lessons for payment, and I used often to sit with him, for he was a very pleasant and intelligent man.[20]

Darwin, coming from a family of committed abolitionists, was a passionate supporter of the anti-slavery campaign. But still, this friendship was unconventional for the times. Many believe that the relationship sowed yet another seed which helped shape the theory of evolution, in which Darwin dismisses arguments that blacks are of an intellectually inferior species to whites.[21]

Darwin joined several of the learned societies which abounded in Edinburgh. He and Grant regularly attended the Wernerian Society, where he heard the great ornithologist John Audubon deliver a paper on the birds of North America. On another occasion, geologist Leonard Horner took Darwin to the Royal Society of Edinburgh, where he was over-awed to see the President, Sir Walter Scott, in the chair. He also attended the Royal Medical Society, but what he heard there seems to have reinforced his dislike of anything medical; his conclusion being that 'Much rubbish was talked there...'[22]

During his specimen-hunting expeditions Darwin befriended fishermen at Newhaven and went on trawling trips with them to add to his collection of specimens:

> [I] made one interesting little discovery... This was that the so-called ova of Flustra had the power of independent movement by means of cilia, and were in fact larvae... I showed that little globular bodies which had been supposed to be the young state

of *Fucus loreus* were the egg-cases of the worm-like *Pontobdella muricata*.[23]

Darwin delivered papers on these discoveries at the Plinian Society, a student forum for presentations and discussions on Natural History which he greatly enjoyed.

By the end of his second year in Edinburgh it was abundantly clear that he was not suited to Medicine. His father now decided that he should become a clergyman, and sent him to Cambridge. Darwin studied Natural Philosophy at Christ's College from 1828 to 1831 under the tutorship of the famous botanist, the Reverend John Henslow. It was Henslow who later recommended Darwin as gentleman companion to Captain Robert Fitzroy on HMS *Beagle,* and so began the well-known story of Darwin's voyage to South America and the Galapagos Islands. Sparked by his observations on Natural History on this trip and developed over the next 20 years, the theory of evolution by natural selection was finally published in *On the Origin of Species* in 1859, when Darwin was 50.[24]

Another celebrated alumnus of the Medical School, novelist Arthur Ignatius Conan Doyle, known world-wide for his fictional private detective Sherlock Holmes, graduated in 1881 and worked as a doctor for 10 years before becoming a full-time writer.

Doyle was born in Edinburgh in 1859, the second child of Irish parents. His father, Charles Doyle, came from an artistic family, but although he had some talent as an illustrator, he struggled to make a living and suffered from bouts of depression which led to drinking; he was institutionalised when Arthur was 20. This family tragedy weighed heavily on Doyle as he grew up. The eldest son, he had a very close relationship with, and felt responsible for, his mother, Mary, whom he called 'the Mam'. Although he was haunted by the fear that he might have inherited his father's constitution, time was to prove otherwise. He attended the Jesuit-run school Stonyhurst College in Lancashire from the age of nine and, while he did not distinguish himself academically, he became an avid reader, made up adventure stories for the younger boys and began to write. But despite the need for an income to support

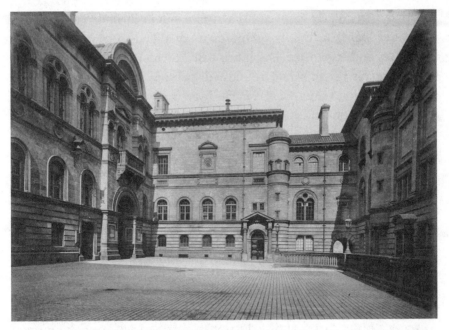

Old Medical School in Teviot Place (the quadrangle of the University New Buildings).

'the Mam' and his siblings, by the time he left school at the age of 16 no decision had been taken on his career.

To make ends meet his mother took in lodgers, one of whom was Bryan Waller, a 22-year-old Edinburgh medical student. Waller persuaded Doyle to follow his example and, obligingly, Doyle passed the University entrance examinations and duly matriculated in Medicine in 1876. At the time the family were living in rented accommodation in Argyle Park Terrace, but they moved to 23 George Square in 1877. Doyle lived comfortably at home while attending lectures in the Medical Faculty, which was by then in the process of moving from 'New College' (now Old College) to a new building in Teviot Place.

As earning money was a priority for Doyle, he served as an outpatient clerk for Dr Joseph Bell at the Infirmary and also carried out periods of locum work at GP practices in Sheffield, Shropshire and Birmingham. Enterprisingly, in 1880 he spent six months as surgeon on the whaler ss *Hope*, bound for the Arctic, where he participated with great enthusiasm in seal and whale hunting.

Doyle particularly enjoyed his assistantship in Birmingham with Dr Reginald Hoare, an Edinburgh graduate qualified to train students in Midwifery and dispensing. Doyle was paid £2 a month for accompanying the doctor on his morning rounds, dispensing in the afternoon and assisting at the evening surgery. He lived with the family, who were of a literary bent, and it was here that he began writing short stories in his spare time. One of these, 'The Mystery of Sasassa Valley', was published in *Chambers' Journal* for a fee of £3.

Doyle never really warmed to his medical studies and although he completed the course he later described it as 'One weary grind at botany, chemistry, anatomy, physiology, and a whole list of compulsory subjects, many of which have a very indirect bearing upon the art of curing.'[25] Nevertheless, he had a keen eye for detail and an excellent memory. Three members of the Medical Faculty – Dr Joseph Bell, Professor Sir Robert Christison and Sir Henry Littlejohn – were used as models for his fictional characters eight years later. Bell was famed for his astute powers of observation and deduction which he used to make instant diagnoses. Doyle 'borrowed' these for Sherlock Holmes. The following example is very evocative of Holmes at his best:

> Bell claimed that he could tell from a man's appearance that he had served, until recently, as a non-commissioned officer in a Highland regiment in Barbados. The surgeon explained his reasoning to his students thus: 'You see, gentlemen, the man was a respectful man but did not remove his hat. They do not in the army, but he would have learned civilian ways had he been long discharged. He had an air of authority and is obviously Scottish. As to Barbados, his complaint is elephantiasis, which is West Indian and not British, and the Scottish regiments are at present in that particular land.'[26]

Christison, whose sphere of influence stretched far beyond the University, was a legendary figure at the time Doyle became a student, not least as the key opponent to women in Medicine; a drama played out just before Doyle enrolled. As Professor of Materia Medica and

Therapeutics from 1832 until 1877, Christison, along with his assistant and successor Professor Thomas Fraser, promoted the study of Pharmacology over Anatomy and Surgery, so that it assumed major significance in the medical curriculum. Both men were in the habit of experimenting with dangerous drugs, including vegetable alkaloids such as cocaine, by using themselves and their students as guinea pigs. On one occasion Christison, known to the students as 'Dignity Bob' because of his 'cold and imperious manner',[27] took a potentially fatal dose of calabar bean (*Physostigma venenosum*), only saving his life by inducing vomiting, but still he was paralysed for several hours. In class Doyle must have been a guinea pig himself on several occasions, and while staying with the Hoares during one of his locums he experimented on himself with tincture of gelseminum (yellow jasmine) which he took regularly for headaches. In the time-honoured manner of his Edinburgh teachers, he took increasing doses of the tincture every night and only stopped at 200 minims (the fatal dose was recorded as 75 minims) because of severe diarrhoea.[28] He then published his findings in the *British Medical Journal* – his first foray into medical publishing.[29] These antics are certainly reminiscent of Holmes, who often experimented in a hospital chemical laboratory to which he had access and had a wide knowledge of poisons – as well as a fondness for cocaine.

Doyle may well have drawn on aspects of Christison's character and actions in creating the austere persona of Holmes and the way in which Christison used his power to influence his colleagues served as a model for Holmes's sinister rival, Professor James Moriarty.

Littlejohn, whose impact as Edinburgh's first Medical Officer of Health is described in Chapter Three, was a medico-legal expert who gave graphic descriptions of recent cases in his popular lectures on Forensic Medicine at one of the extra-mural schools. From him Doyle learnt how scientific advances, such as photography and fingerprinting, now accepted as evidence in the courts, were being used to apprehend criminals. It was exactly this link between modern scientific discoveries and solving crimes that Doyle exploited with such success in his Holmes novels.

Doyle, who later described himself as a student as being 'one of the

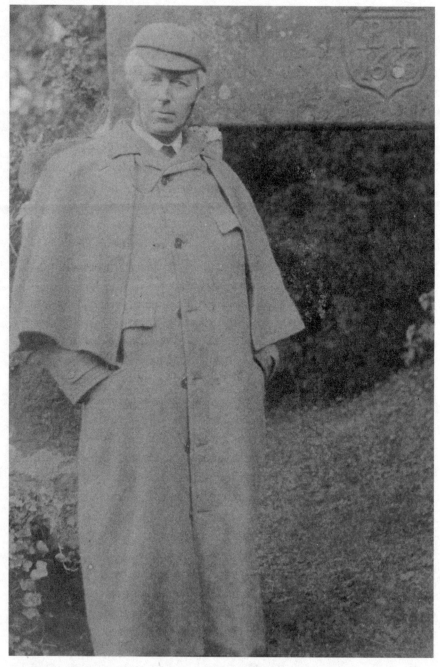

Portrait of Joseph Bell, the inspiration behind Sherlock Holmes.

ruck, neither lingering nor gaining – a 60 per cent man at examinations',[30] gained his medical degree in 1881. Despite the urgent need to earn a living, he still had no plans for his future career. To bide time he enrolled for another stint as a ship's doctor, this time with the African Steamship Company on the ss *Mayumba*, bound for West Africa. For looking after the medical needs of the 30 passengers Doyle was paid £12 a month, the whole round trip lasting three months.

On his return Doyle was invited to join a student friend, George Budd, who had recently set up in general practice in Plymouth. Budd offered free consultations, making a living by charging for the drugs which his wife prepared and he liberally prescribed. Doyle fell in with this for a while but the two were soon arguing and Doyle, now using the name Conan Doyle (Conan was his paternal grandmother's maiden name), moved to Portsmouth to set up on his own. He stayed there for seven years, supplementing the living he made through his practice with income from selling short stories to the many periodicals of the day. Although there is no clear record of the cases he studied, during this period he must have written his MD thesis on syphilis: *An Essay Upon the Vasomotor Changes in Tabes Dorsalis*, since he returned to Edinburgh for his degree ceremony just before his wedding in 1885.

At the time of his marriage to Louise Hawkins, the sister of a patient who had died of meningitis, Doyle was feeling dissatisfied with his alternative career in writing. He wrote short stories with amazing energy and speed, many of which were eventually published, but he had not found his literary voice or identified his preferred genre. However, perhaps due to a more settled home life after his marriage, within a year he had decided to use his medical and scientific expertise in the up-and-coming genre of the detective novel, a vital step in his transformation from jobbing doctor to famous novelist.

Doyle began his first Sherlock Holmes novel, *A Study in Scarlet*, in 1886. He seems to have plucked the names of the main players, as well as their characters, from among his friends and acquaintances. Holmes came from the famous North American physician and best-selling author, Oliver Wendell Holmes, whom Doyle much admired; and the name of Holmes' companion, Dr John Watson, probably came from Doyle's fellow GP in Southsea, Dr James Watson, an Edinburgh graduate who had practised in China. After some hawking around, the novel was eventually published in its entirety in *Beeton's Christmas Annual* for 1887, for a fee of £25. It was an instant success.

Doyle did not abandon his medical career immediately. After a chance meeting with Vernon Ford, a surgeon from the Portsmouth Eye and Ear Hospital, he undertook some part-time work in the eye department and decided to specialise in opthalmology. He was advised to spend a period of time studying the eye in Vienna and then to try his luck as an eye specialist in London, and so he and Louise, now with baby daughter Mary Louise, travelled to Vienna in January 1891. Here he attended a course at the University, hastily writing stories between lectures to earn their keep. By the end of March they were in London, living in a rented house in Montague Place, Bloomsbury, and Doyle found a consulting room in the private doctors' enclave of Upper Wimpole Street. This was the breakthrough; not *for* his medical career, but *because* of it. He had decided to embark upon a series of stories starring Sherlock Holmes. He wrote 'A Scandal in Bohemia', the first Holmes story to be published in *Strand* magazine, 'in his new Upper Wimpole Street consulting room, and was able to do so because, as an unknown quantity, he had no patients.[31] The publisher liked the story and was keen for more of the same. In a flurry of activity Doyle had completed three more Holmes stories by May 1891 when the literary flow was interrupted by a severe bout of the flu. It was during this episode of enforced bed rest that he reviewed his life and later wrote:

> I determined with a wild rush of joy to cut the painter and to trust for ever to my power of writing [realising that] I should at last be my own master. No longer would I have to conform to professional dress or try to please any one else. I would be free to live how I liked and where I liked. It was one of the great moments of exaltation of my life.[32]

Doyle never again practised Medicine on a regular basis, although on two occasions later in life his medical training came in useful.

In late 1899, for patriotic reasons, but also perhaps to seek some relief from his wife's illness (she was suffering from TB and eventually died in 1906), Doyle joined the staff of the Langman Hospital, a privately funded, 100-bed, tented hospital, heading for South Africa. The aim was to assist the new Royal Medical Corps to cope with casualties from the Boer War. By the time the hospital team reached Cape Town in March 1900 the Boers were already in retreat, but the tents were pitched on the Ramblers cricket ground at the recently relieved Bloemfontein in Orange Free State. Here Doyle became rather busier than he had expected because of a typhoid epidemic which broke out after the Boers cut off the town's water supply, forcing the occupants to use contaminated water from old wells and the river Modder.

Doyle's second return to Medicine, in 1906, involved the case of lawyer George Edalji, which was fictionalised by novelist Julian Barnes in *Arthur and George*.[33] Edalji was the son of the Indian vicar in the village of Great Wyrley, Staffordshire, who had been convicted of the extraordinary crime of mutilating sheep, cows and horses in the village. A popular campaign against the verdict had procured his release from prison after serving three years of a seven-year sentence, but had not gained him a pardon. When Doyle met Edalji he immediately deduced by the way he read the newspaper that he had astigmatism, a diagnosis that was confirmed by an optician. Doyle concluded that, with his poor eyesight, Edalji could not have carried out crimes perpetrated in fields at dead of night. Doyle was satisfied that the accusation was false and racially motivated. His high-profile interest in the case revitalised the campaign to establish Edalji's innocence and he was eventually exonerated. This case is said to have influenced the argument for the establishment of the Court of Criminal Appeal in 1907.

Oddly for a man with a medical training who prided himself (as did his fictional detective) on his powers of logical scientific deduction, Doyle embraced spiritualism, after considering the idea for many years. By the time he died of heart failure at the age of 71, he had already devised his own spiritualist funeral service. At his memorial service in the Albert Hall the medium Estelle Robert assured the crowd of 6,000 that Doyle was among them.

Doyle was an immensely popular figure in his time and remains so today. His invention of consulting detective Sherlock Holmes has certainly gained him a place in literary history alongside other early crime writers who shaped the genre, such as Wilkie Collins and Edgar Allan Poe. A statue commemorating the man and his work stands in Picardy Place, Edinburgh, where he was born.

CHAPTER 6
Eminent Physicians

THE 19TH CENTURY was not only a time for improvements in medical practice but also one of groundbreaking advances in the understanding of disease. The Edinburgh Medical School played a significant role in training doctors who became renowned for their descriptions of the pathology of some common and deadly diseases. The understanding they gained served to shape future treatments and the knowledge and insight garnered by these early medical pioneers remains relevant to Medicine today.

During the first half of the century medical experts clashed over whether treating symptoms, rather than investigating the cause of disease, was paramount in ensuring the best patient care. This included James Syme, who derided the use of pathology and pushed for its Chair to be abolished, and James Young Simpson who, by contrast, fervently supported the need to integrate pathology into medical teaching and practice. The critics of pathology were eventually silenced by evidence of the benefits of post-mortem to study 'gross anatomy', and microscopy that revealed pathological changes, enabling the process of disease to be categorised, for instance as inflammatory, malignant or degenerative in nature.

Medical alumni from Edinburgh forged ahead in the greater understanding of disease by characterising and describing various conditions. John Hughes Bennett gained fame for being the first to describe leukaemia, while other Edinburgh graduates had the conditions

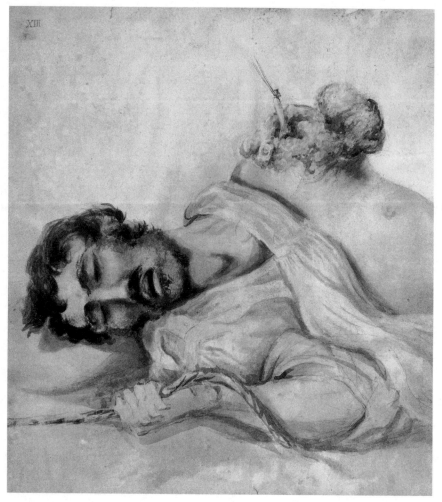

Detail from a watercolour of a wounded soldier at Waterloo by Charles Bell.

they characterised named after them. They included Richard Bright with Bright's Disease – now known as glomerulonephritis; Thomas Addison with Addison's Disease – adrenal failure – and Addison's (Pernicious) Anaemia; Thomas Hodgkin with Hodgkin's Lymphoma and Charles Bell with Bell's Palsy.

Charles Bell was born in 1774 and was the younger brother of John Bell, who is regarded as the founder of Applied Surgical Anatomy.[1] The brothers were from a family of six children and Charles was the youngest. Despite the same surname, they were not related to the dynasty of surgeons headed up by Benjamin Bell. John was 11 years senior to Charles and no doubt took on a somewhat paternal role as their father, an Episcopalian clergyman, had passed away five years after Charles was born. Although John studied Surgical Anatomy under the esteemed Monro secundus, he felt that his tutor lacked any first-hand knowledge of surgical problems. To this end John taught Anatomy while also practising as a surgeon and was among the first to emphasise the relevance of anatomy to surgical practice. At the age of 18, Charles became his apprentice and was soon delivering lectures to a class of more than 100 students.[2]

The pair were elected members of the Royal College of Surgeons of Edinburgh, but this did not mean that all doors were open to them. As was commonly the case in Edinburgh medical circles at the time, rivalries and disputes seemed to overshadow their careers. John Bell provoked jealousy by his success and alienated some contemporaries with outspoken criticism of the unnecessary pain and suffering inflicted by incompetent surgeons. When the Professor of Medicine, James Gregory, persuaded the authorities that only six members of the College of Surgeons should act as Surgeons to the Royal Infirmary, each for a period of two years,[3] the brothers were, in effect, banished from surgical practice in the hospital. John decided to stay in Edinburgh and went on to find fame as a teacher, surgeon and author of textbooks on human Anatomy and Surgery but Charles, who was to become renowned for his work on the nervous system, resolved to forge his career in London. On his arrival there, a fellow surgeon told him that if he had experienced difficulties in Edinburgh he would find more in London.[4]

Not one to give up easily, Charles found ways to make ends meet. Brought up by his artist mother to develop wide cultural interests, he was a gifted artist and delivered lectures to artists and medical students in a dilapidated house where he also practised Medicine. His *Essay on the Anatomy of Expression in Painting* (1806 with an expanded edition in 1824) gained him attention. On hearing that Queen Victoria had a copy, he exclaimed, 'Oh happiness in the extreme! that I should ever write anything fit to be dirtied by her snuffy fingers.'[5]

Charles was fascinated by the nervous system. On establishing that all nerves have two roots – dorsal and ventral – leading to and from the spinal cord, he stimulated these individually, using a donkey as an experimental animal. His findings that an irritation of the 'ventral root caused cramps, while a disturbance of the dorsal root produced no visible symptoms', suggested that the two nerve roots had different functions. His radical conclusions were published in 1811 in his *New Idea of the Anatomy of the Brain*, but the book did not gain much notice, perhaps because it was privately printed in an edition limited to 100 copies. However, two years later Charles was invited to become a member of the Royal College of Surgeons of England and the following year he was elected as surgeon at London's Middlesex Hospital.

With his enthusiasm for surgery, he viewed the Battle of Waterloo in 1815 as an opportunity to use his operating skills. He made his way to Brussels – without a passport – and treated the wounded from morning until night by which time 'his clothes were stiff with blood' and his arm 'powerless with the exertion of using the knife'.[6] He also sketched and painted what he saw. Some of his works of art are still on display at the Royal College of Surgeons of Edinburgh.

On his return to London, Charles turned his focus once more to the nervous system and was appointed Professor of Anatomy and Surgery to the English Royal College of Surgeons in 1824. *The Nervous System of the Human Body* (1830), in which he expands on his *New Idea*, distinguishes clearly between sensory nerves, which conduct impulses such as touch and pain to the central nervous system, and motor nerves, which convey messages from the brain or other nerve centres to organs such as muscles, which cause them to contract. This observation, which was confirmed experimentally and more fully elaborated 11 years later by the French physiologist François Magendie, became known as Bell's Law or the Bell-Magendie Law. There was some controversy as to which man first made this discovery, but Charles was certainly the first person to describe the paralysis resulting from a lesion of the facial nerve, now known as Bell's Palsy.

His work was revolutionary in contesting the prevailing theory that

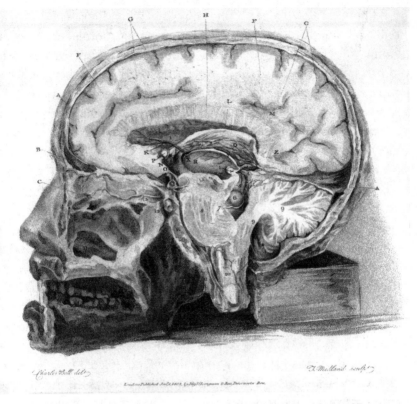

Section of the brain from Bell's *The Anatomy of the Brain Explained in a Series of Engravings.*

all nerves were ostensibly the same. According to this theory, the reason the retina conveyed light to the brain, while skin conveyed touch or pain, was because the retina was more sensitive than skin. Charles argued that if this were true, the pain of a needle touching the retina would be such that 'life could not bear so great a pain'; whereas instead, the needle gives a 'sensation of a spark of fire'.[7]

Although he spent most of his career in London, Charles was to return to the city of his alma mater. Despite his high renown in London and a large surgical practice, he felt that the capital was 'a place to live in, but not to die in'[8] and at the age of 61 left to take up the Chair in Surgery at Edinburgh. He was to die while visiting a friend in Worcester six years later.

Like Charles Bell, three later medical students at the University of Edinburgh also gained fame applying what they had learned in Edinburgh south of the border. Although this contingent of medical alumni – Richard Bright, Thomas Addison and Thomas Hodgkin – did not study in Edinburgh at exactly the same time, they all became eminent doctors at Guy's Hospital in London, with careers that were inextricably linked. Throughout their professional lives, it would not have been uncommon for them to work collaboratively or refer to each other's cases and both Bright and Addison were to hold the elevated post as the hospital Physician at Guy's.

Bright started his studies in Edinburgh in 1808, Addison in 1812 and Hodgkin in 1820. They came from very different backgrounds: Bright, brought up in Bristol, was a son of a merchant banker; Addison, from near Newcastle-upon-Tyne, was the son of a grocer; and Hodgkin was brought up in a Quaker family in London. In deciding to study in Edinburgh, Bright may well have favoured quality over tradition. For Addison the decision was more likely to have hinged on financial considerations, and Hodgkin, as a Quaker, would have been declined access to ecclesiastical seats of learning such as Oxford or Cambridge.

Bright, the first of the three to graduate, completed his degree with a thesis, *On Contagious Erysipelas*, in which he stressed the infectious nature of this skin condition and its similarities to puerperal fever. When he took up the post as Assistant Physician at Guy's in 1820 it was clear that he had a gift for making meticulous clinical observations. He followed his observations up with equally thorough post-mortem examinations and was keen to use scientific techniques to back up his clinical observations. One such method – detecting protein in urine by heating a sample in a spoon to see if the liquid became opaque before boiling – served to establish his hypothesis that body swelling, or dropsy, and the presence of the protein albumin in the urine were clinical signs of severe kidney disease. Making this connection secured his reputation as a physician, and the disease became known as Bright's Disease, although it is now called glomerulonephritis. The practice-based teaching at Edinburgh had such an impact on him that he made certain his students also gained extensive practical experience in addition to attending lectures on theory.[9]

Bright was promoted to Physician at Guy's in 1824, where he remained until his retirement in 1843, after which he carried on with his medical practice until his death from heart failure at the age of 69.

When Bright retired from Guy's, it was Addison who succeeded him as the hospital's Physician, just as he had previously succeeded him in the role of Assistant Physician. Addison had qualified at Edinburgh in 1815 with a thesis *Concerning Syphilis and Mercury* and although he subsequently held a number of posts in London and was a fully qualified physician, he started out at Guy's as a physician's pupil. This was not to set him back and he quickly rose up the ranks, with responsibilities that included sharing the post of Lecturer on Practical Medicine at Guy's with Bright, becoming the sole incumbent when Bright stepped down from this role in 1840.

Despite the high regard with which he was held as a physician, Addison came across as somewhat austere. This may have been down to shyness and an aversion to boasting of his achievements, but by all accounts he was a brilliant lecturer, attracting large crowds of students. His demeanour instilled respect among his students, as one by the name of Wilks confirms:

The force of his words was enhanced by his mode of delivery and by the presence of the man himself... His penetrating glance seemed to look through you, and his whole demeanour was that of a leader of men, enhanced by his somewhat martial attitude.[10]

Addison's interest in skin diseases led to the description of two diseases, both named after him: Addison's (Pernicious) Anaemia and Addison's Disease. In 1849 he published a paper in the *Medical Gazette* describing a fatal anaemia of unknown cause in which the patient's skin becomes 'more and more bloodless' and has 'some resemblance to a bad wax figure'.[11] Although he at first linked this anaemia to the destruction of the adrenal gland he found by chance in his first patient, he later refuted this and the cause remained unknown for around a hundred years. In 1920 a diet of raw liver was found to be an effective treatment, but it was not until 1948 that the active ingredient in liver, vitamin B12, was isolated and pernicious anaemia shown to be caused by a B12 deficiency. Addison's second discovery – Addison's Disease – was published in a monograph in 1855, in which he described the symptoms of 11 patients:

> The leading and characteristic features of the morbid state to which I direct your attention, are, anaemia, general languor and debility, remarkable feebleness of the heart action, irritability of the stomach, and a peculiar change of colour in the skin, occurring in connexion with a diseased condition of the 'supra-renal capsules'.[12]

Again anaemia was among the key features, but as a skin specialist, it was the bronzing of the skin which Addison first noticed:

> a dingy or smoky appearance, of various tints or shades of deep amber or chestnut-brown; and in one instant the skin was so universally and so deeply darkened, that, but for his features, the patient might have been mistaken for a mulatto. [13]

On post-mortem examination Addison found that the supra-renal capsule, now called the adrenal gland, had been destroyed in all cases, either by TB or cancer. We now know that the adrenal glands produce the vital hormone cortisone, a lack of which causes Addison's Disease and is fatal if left untreated.

Despite the mark Addison made on Medicine, perhaps because of his unwillingness for self-promotion, the only medical journal to carry his obituary was the *Medical Times and Gazette*, which had also published his description of Addison's Disease:

> We believe that Dr Addison has made a discovery which is one of the most important practical medicine has produced for many years, and one in every way worthy of the untiring zeal and energy in professional pursuits which have characterised his life.[14]

Compared to Bright and Addison, Hodgkin's career was dogged by disappointment. Despite the importance of identifying a novel malignancy of lymph nodes, career progression at Guy's was restricted due to friction with the hospital treasurer and he was passed over for the post of Assistant Physician when Addison was promoted to full Physician in 1837. Although he was invited to share the Assistant Physician post with another doctor, he would have been the more junior of the two and refused. Having left Guy's greatly disillusioned, he became Director of the Museum and lecturer in the Theory and Practice of Medicine at St Thomas's Medical School in 1842. This again was to bring disappointment, as he was replaced after two years when the Faculty was reorganised, placing emphasis on lecturers' popularity with the students. His personal life was also dealt a blow when he was forbidden to marry his first cousin, Sarah Godlee, such a union being frowned upon by Quakers. He even wrote a pamphlet citing theological and scientific evidence that there was little risk in such a relationship, publicly opposing the Society of Friends' rule, but to no avail.[15]

Unlike Bright and Addison, Hodgkin had originally set out on a career to become an apothecary. As a young man he worked as assistant to a William Allen (a family friend who lectured at Guy's and sold medicines to other apothecaries), and at the apothecary shop of his mother's cousin, John Glaisyer, in Brighton. It soon became apparent that it was not so much the business side of the shop he enjoyed but the practice of Medicine. This, coupled with restrictions placed upon apothecaries, no doubt influenced his decision to become a doctor. Even though the 1815 Medical Reform Act (Apothecaries Act) legalised the practice of Medicine by apothecaries – before this law was passed apothecaries could only charge for the medicines sold and not for advice given – they were generally viewed as tradesmen and their professional advancement was limited.[16] While an apothecary surgeon could join the Royal College of Surgeons as a member, there was little chance of becoming a Fellow.

At the age of 21, Hodgkin announced his intentions to become a physician. He stayed in London for a year, attending lectures at Guy's, before heading north to Edinburgh. The journey in 1820 was made by boat and took four days, during which he was seasick throughout. It cost £10 to matriculate at the University and Hodgkin also paid £4 4s to the professor of each course he took[17] but he was disappointed with some of his lectures. Writing home, he described Dr Francis Home, the University's first lecturer in Materia Medica, as clever and agreeable but whose lecture was almost an exact repetition of another lecturer, though not as audible.[18]

Hodgkin was a humble young man and when he presented a medical paper entitled *On the Uses of the Spleen* to the Royal Society of Edinburgh during his first year in Edinburgh, he prefaced it by acknowledging that he might be attacked for presumption in even tackling the subject.[19] However, his realisation that the spleen and the lymph nodes were somehow functionally linked was a prelude to his later research.

During his studies in Edinburgh, Hodgkin took time out in Paris to widen his medical knowledge. Here, post-mortem examination was viewed as an extension of clinical teaching and great emphasis was placed on pathology to gain insight into how the body works in health and disease, to improve diagnosis and to classify disease processes. Contemporaries in Paris included Robert Knox, who had arranged for a separate dissecting room at the Pitié-Salpêtrière Hospital and Hodgkin was one of those invited to share it to study pathologic anatomy by dissection.[20] While in France he was also introduced to the stethoscope, a simple wooden tube resembling an ear trumpet invented in Paris in 1816 by René Laënnec. On his return to Britain, Hodgkin addressed the Physical Society at Guy's on what he believed to be the 'first introduction of mediate austiculation to a London School'. His talk included suggestions about the length and the kind of wood to be used for the cylinder and its role in diagnosing conditions such as tuberculosis.[21] Absent-mindedly, Hodgkin left the stethoscope behind in London when he returned to Edinburgh but fortunately it was soon forwarded to him. His thesis focused on the absorptive mechanisms within the body, encompassing the absorption of air by the lungs, the lymphatic system and the veins.

After graduation and further travels in Europe, Hodgkin took up a post at the London Dispensary in 1825, treating the poor, and an unpaid position as clinical clerk at Guy's Hospital. In 1826 he was appointed to the combined post of Inspector of the Dead and Curator of the Museum at Guy's. These two roles suited his interest in Pathology, fostered in Edinburgh and Paris. However, as Knox had found with regards to the supply of bodies in Edinburgh, obtaining and preserving anatomical specimens was frowned upon in some quarters. During one of a number of autopsies that Hodgkin performed for Bright, in which he was asked to preserve the kidneys, spleen, liver and heart, he was advised to arrive for the post-mortem surreptitiously.[22]

Hodgkin broke the mould of traditional lectures in 1827 when he gave a course of lectures on Pathology – the first such course of its kind in England. But despite the innovative subject, his highly intellectual style was not always popular with students who were not required to attend to pass their examinations. In 1832, he first described the disease which now bears his name, Hodgkin's Disease or Hodgkin's Lymphoma, in a lecture to the Medical and Chirurgical Society.

Hodgkin focused on an abnormality of the lymph glands – the so-called absorbent glands within the body – detailing a series of cases of enlargement of the glands which was not secondary to tumours or inflammation and involved all the lymph glands as well as the spleen. Publication of his observations soon followed in the society's journal: 'On Some Morbid Appearances of the Absorbent Glands and Spleen' describes seven cases, most of which were from Guy's under the care of Bright and Addison.

Hodgkin held to his Quaker beliefs throughout his life, and after leaving Guy's and St Thomas's devoted his life to the needs of the poor and mentally ill. He became a physician at the London Cutaneous Infirmary, later known as the Hospital for the Diseases of the Skin, as well as a medical officer for the National Provident Institute, both Quaker establishments. He began eventually to withdraw from Medicine and spent much time travelling. He died on a trip to Israel in Jaffa in 1866.

The reputation of men such as Bright, Addison and Hodgkin no doubt served to enhance the prestige of an Edinburgh medical education. However not everyone chose to apply what they had learned in Edinburgh south of the border. John Hughes Bennett, who enrolled at the University in 1833, stayed on in the city where he rose to the ranks of Professor and became famed for his description of leukaemia.

Prior to starting his medical degree, Bennett had spent time apprenticed to a surgeon in Kent. Like Bright, Addison and Hodgkin, he displayed a strong interest in Pathology and during his apprenticeship had assisted in post-mortem examinations. He was an excellent student and as well as applying himself to his studies was elected president of both the Royal Medical Society and the Royal Physical Society and was vice-president of the Anatomical and Physiological Society. He was awarded a gold medal for best clinical report of surgical cases on Professor Sir James Syme's wards.

Sir Charles Bell also recommended that Bennett's thesis, *The Physiology and Pathology of the Brain: Being an Attempt to Ascertain what Portions of that Organ are More Immediately Connected with Motion, Sensation and Intelligence*, be awarded a medal. Bennett was later informed by Syme that he would have received a second medal, had there not been a rule that two medals could not be awarded to the same competitor.[23]

He extended his medical education with a trip to the Continent, spending two years in Paris and visiting universities, including Heidelberg and Berlin, before returning to Edinburgh in 1841 where he gave extra-mural lectures on Histology, Physiology, Pathology and the diagnosis of disease. Bennett would use the microscope to illustrate his talks as well as running private courses, limited to no more than six students, on the 'Practical Manipulation of the Microscope'. These were the first of their kind in the UK. His obituary in the *British Medical Journal* read:

> The clear, precise, methodological style pursued by the French physicians harmonised with his own qualities of mind, and there is little doubt the system of clinical instruction which he afterwards successfully introduced into Edinburgh, was carefully elaborated by him while in Paris.[24]

However his efforts to introduce Histology into medical education received a mixed reception. In the following winter session he had five students and by the summer he only had three and had to abandon his course. Only four out of between 50 and 60 members of the University's medical staff took up an invitation to attend his lectures.[25]

In 1842 Bennett was appointed a fellow of the Royal College of Physicians of Edinburgh and the Royal Society of Edinburgh. He subsequently took on the role of Physician to the Royal Dispensary and Pathologist to the Royal Infirmary of Edinburgh and also became a University Lecturer in Medicine. His students gained practical experience, under supervision, in examining and prescribing for patients. In 1848, he was appointed as Chair of the Institutes of Medicine. Despite the initially lukewarm reaction to his teachings on the microscope, Bennett continued to extol its virtues. In May 1845, when giving an introductory address to a course of lectures on Histology and the use of the microscope, he stated:

The microscope, long looked upon as a source of amusement and as affording to the rich an elegant pastime, is daily found to become more useful in the sciences and arts... In short, its practical applications are daily extending; but in no science does it bid fair to be so eminently useful as that in medicine...

In Pathology, how vague are the ideas attached to inflammation, softening of the tubercles and other morbid processes. On these a flood of light has been thrown by the microscope. This subject, indeed, has been comparatively little studied, and yet I know of none which is likely to yield such interesting and important results to a microscopic inquirer. The apathy of the profession, however, on this point, has hitherto been most singular.[26]

By encouraging the use of the microscope, Bennett was also promoting the role of scientific investigation in medical research. As discussed elsewhere in this book, this was sometimes seen as a challenge to established principles whereby patients were treated on the basis of observed symptoms. In 1865 Bennett's surgical colleague Syme urged

...against paying undue attention to the system of minute investigation at present so much in fashion. I am no enemy to the microscope, and on the contrary, believe that much useful as well as curious information may be obtained through its assistance; but I beg to remind you that the utmost amount of knowledge derived from this source can never supply the want of acquaintance with the form, structure, and relations of parts, which are obvious to the unaided senses of sight and touch.[27]

However the microscope was of key importance in Bennett's investigations into the disease now known as leukaemia. The story began when an Edinburgh physician, David Craigie, became intrigued by the clinical presentation of a patient, Peter Campbell, who was admitted to the hospital in 1841 with severe lethargy, an enlarged spleen and lymph glands. The patient later died. When another patient, John Monteith, also died with a splenic tumour and similar symptoms, Craigie felt that the two men must share the same 'internal and pathological state'. Bennett was called upon to carry out the post-mortem examination on Monteith and reported his findings in a paper entitled 'Case of Hypertrophy of the Spleen and Liver in which Death Took Place from Suppuration of the Blood', which was published in 1845 in the *Edinburgh Medical and Surgical Journal* alongside Craigie's report on Campbell's case.[28]

What Bennett saw in the blood of the patient both amazed and confused him. Previously it was known that a focus of infection or inflammation in the body may cause an increase in white blood cells and, as these are the cells that form pus, this was described as 'pus cells in the blood'. In Monteith's case the blood was so 'full of pus' that it was pale in colour, but no focus of infection could be found. Under the microscope Bennett identified the abnormal white cells which we now know to be the malignant cells of leukaemia, literally meaning 'white blood'. In his paper Bennett left the reader with the questions, 'Were the corpuscles contained in the blood really those of pus? And if so, how were they produced?'

In the same year Rudolf Virchow, at the Charité Hospital in Berlin, also reported a case of leukaemia in a 50-year-old female patient. Virchow's '*Weisses Blut*' ('White Blood') was published six weeks after Bennett's paper and was not as detailed.[29] The debate that arose as to prior claim was not so much between Virchow and Bennett, but rather one that was stirred up by other members of the medical profession. However Virchow himself resolved the question in 1858, stating publicly that Bennett had 'observed a case of indubitable leukaemia some months before I saw my first case'.

Bennett, whose father was a theatre impresario and mother an actress, was not shy of taking centre-stage and often made contentious interventions into medical debates, bloodletting being a case in point. While historically this had been a common form of medical treatment, during the 1830s its use – particularly in managing acute inflammations such as pneumonia – was in decline.[30] Some physicians insisted that the reason for this was merely that bloodletting was intended for 'sthenic' conditions – involving agitation and fever – but that it was now more common for patients to display an 'asthenic' type of disease, where they were weak and required nourishment rather than bloodletting. One theory gained currency that it was not so much the disease but the human body itself that had altered to an asthenic type that could no longer withstand bloodletting.[31]

Bennett stepped into the debate in 1857. His contention was that bloodletting was no longer appropriate, and never had been; he used statistics to demonstrate that bloodletting increased mortality rates, with one in three cases of profuse bleeding being followed by death while, according to his own records, only four patients out of 129 who received 'restorative' treatment had died.[32] The attention given to his controversial claim that laboratory science indicated that bloodletting was bad for the patient effectively gave him a platform from which to promote his own agenda of advancing Pathology. [33] He found a heavyweight opponent in Edinburgh's eminent Professor of Medicine, William Pulteney Alison, the leader of the Scottish medical establishment, who took the view that while laboratory science might help explain therapeutic activity, it should not direct it.[34] Citing clinical experience and learned traditions, Alison proclaimed that bloodletting

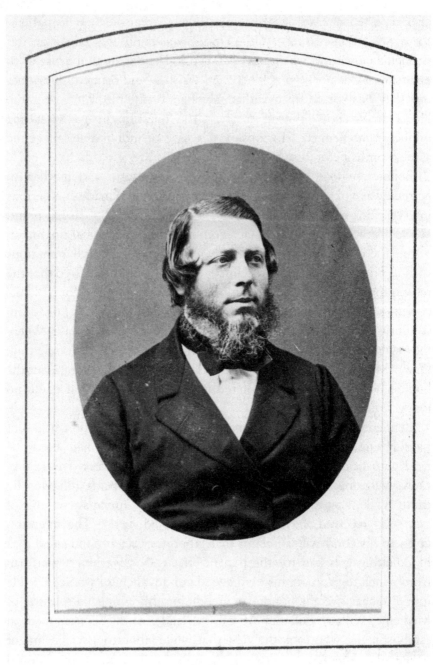

John Hughes Bennett.

produced 'favourable subjective manifestations that, together, indicated the very nature of its efficacy.'[35]

The debate was well reported in the medical press. It spread across the Atlantic, with most in the mainstream of the medical profession aligning themselves with Alison. Those practising more unorthodox and alternative treatments jumped on the Bennett bandwagon, doing little to serve his cause or enhance his reputation. The wrangle was not quickly resolved and as late as 1892, the eminent Canadian physician William Osler wrote in *The Principles and Practice of Medicine*:

> During the first five decades of this century the profession bled too much, but during the last five decades we have certainly bled too little. Pneumonia is one of the diseases in which a timely bleed may save life.[36]

Retrospectively Bennett is seen as having done more than anyone to end excessive bleeding as a routine method of treatment.[37] As his obituary in the *British Medical Journal* anticipated:

> When all the controversies with which his name is associated will have been forgotten, the important services which he rendered to practical medicine will be even more highly appreciated than they are at present.[38]

Bennett's contribution to Medicine was recognised by the University of Edinburgh in 1901 – 26 years after his death – when it opened a laboratory bearing his name, following a donation from one of his daughters. Although the original laboratory no longer exists, a new John Hughes Bennett Laboratory was opened in 1998 by the University at the Western General Hospital site, in collaboration with the Leukaemia Research Fund, UK (now Leukaemia and Lymphoma Research); it relocated to the Queen's Medical Research Institute in 2007.

CHAPTER 7

Modern Times

IN EDINBURGH, MEDICAL pioneers have continued to make their mark with advances over the last century. These have included the UK's first kidney transplant, a revolutionary treatment for tuberculosis, a synthetic vaccine for hepatitis B and the cloning of Dolly the Sheep. The distinguishing feature of the Edinburgh experience has been that teaching, research and medical care have always gone hand-in-glove. Today, around 250 students graduate each year in Medicine at Edinburgh, one of the most competitive courses for places in the UK. The Medical School was also rated top in Britain for hospital, based clinical subjects in the 2008 Government Funding Councils' research assessment exercise.

General Practice
In the 20th century the medical landscape was dramatically changed with the introduction of the National Health Service (NHS) in 1948. Edinburgh led the way in training medical students in General Practice as well as recognising the importance of nursing by setting up the UK's first Department of Nursing Studies.

When the NHS was introduced, with the ethos of free healthcare for all, public dispensaries that had previously provided treatment for patients who could not afford to see a private doctor were shut down. The end of public dispensaries created a void for the training of doctors in primary care. Dr Richard Scott of the University's Department of Public

Health and Social Science set up a general medical practice to provide this training for the medical students, based on the following analysis:

> It was obvious, therefore, that if the Medical School wished to salvage any of the teaching facilities which were offered by the old dispensary system, it might well have to become involved in the provision to a group of patients, of medical care at least comparable in respect both of quality and quantity with that offered by any general practitioner within the framework of the Health Service.[1]

The initiative was originally run as an experiment at the Royal Dispensary, West Richmond Street, which dated back to 1783. By 1951 around 30 medical students received three months' training at the Teaching General Practice Unit, which included visits to patients' homes as well as consulting room examinations. The number of students was limited by the need to establish what the University referred to as a 'secure and continuing' doctor–patient relationship. In 1952 a grant from the Rockefeller Foundation enabled the University to extend training in general practice to more students by opening a second centre in the Cowgate at the site of the Livingstone Memorial Dispensary.

By 1956 each practice, with a staff of two doctors, one nurse, a medico-social worker and a secretary, was providing medical care for around 2,500 registered patients. The Unit became the world's first university Department of General Practice and, in 1963, Scott was appointed to the Chair of Medicine in Relation to General Practice, a position then unique in the UK. Today the department is known as Community Health Sciences – General Practice, and is based at 20 West Richmond Street. It delivers more than 12 per cent of clinical teaching within the Edinburgh medical curriculum, with research topics including cancer, allergy and respiratory disease, palliative care, e-health and primary mental health care.

Nursing Studies

Not only was the University of Edinburgh at the forefront of training

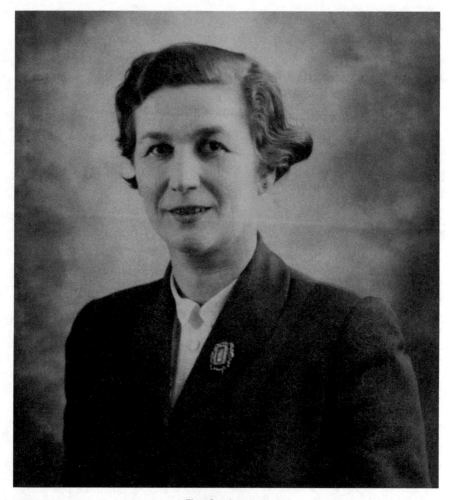

Elsie Stephenson.

doctors, but it was also the first UK university to set up a Nursing Teaching Unit in 1956. Not long after opening, the Nursing Teaching Unit's name was changed to Nursing Studies Unit after the University Court ruled that this would be 'more appropriate to a unit which is concerned not merely with the training of teachers, but with the research and courses for leaders in the field of nursing'.[2]

The unit was headed by Elsie Stephenson, a trained nurse, midwife and health visitor who was keen to improve education and research opportunities for nurses. During the war she was Senior Sister with the Joint War Organisation of the British Red Cross Society and Order of St John of Jerusalem. The position took her to refugee camps in Egypt and northern Italy and in Germany she was Acting Matron of a sanatorium. In Yugoslavia she worked in a public health nursing service and in Berlin was a member of a child welfare team surveying health, nutrition and welfare services. After the war had ended she was also involved in organising Red Cross centres in Singapore and conducted a survey of child welfare conditions in British North Borneo, Brunei and Sarawak.[3]

The *Nursing Times* warmly welcomed the opening of the unit and the appointment of Stephenson as its head:

Nurses will rejoice at this significant first appointment of a nurse as a member of the Faculty of a British University, especially as the appointment as advertised was not limited to nurses.[4]

Those who enrolled as students completed an 18-month course to graduate as nurse-tutors with studies including Psychology, biblical Studies, Social Anthropology, Economic Geography and Moral Philosophy. The first cohort of 13 students – two of them men – received their diplomas in 1958. Two years later, nursing students enrolled at Edinburgh were also able to study for a degree. The programme lasted five years and students graduated in Arts or Science before their final qualification in Nursing. The move led the *Sunday Post* to run the headline – 'Gosh – The Nurse Has Got an MA!'[5] Demand was so strong it inspired a headline in the *Edinburgh Evening Dispatch*, 'Nurses in "Queue" for University Course.'[6] Work within the unit included research into nursing methods and patient attitudes to hospitals and nurses. When it became the Department of Nursing Studies, Muriel Powell, matron of St George's Hospital in London, commented in the ninth *Nursing Mirror* Lecture, in 1967:

In accepting nursing studies as a department within the University, Edinburgh has done for nursing in the 1960s what Florence Nightingale did for nursing in Britain just over 100 years ago.[7]

Stephenson had a very international perspective, perhaps because of her experiences during the war, and this led her to found the *International Journal of Nursing Studies* in 1964. That same year the first students enrolled at Edinburgh's new International School of Advanced Nursing Studies, which was set up in collaboration with the World Health Organisation. On completion of a year-long course, graduate nurses received a diploma and non-graduates a certificate.

Stephenson died in post in 1967, at the age of 51, and the directorship of the Department of Nursing Studies was taken up by Margaret Scott Wright, a History graduate from Edinburgh, the following year. Her background had included working as a research assistant at Unilever before training as a nurse and then qualifying as a midwife as well as completing a phd at Edinburgh's Department of Nursing Studies. Roles as Deputy Matron at St George's Hospital in London and matron of the Middlesex Hospital Teaching Group in London also meant that she was no stranger to responsibility.

Four years later the University set up a Nursing Research Unit with funds from the Scottish Home and Health Department. Its remit was to research the needs of the Health Service in Scotland. The next year, Wright was appointed to the first Chair of Nursing Studies in the UK in what was again seen as a groundbreaking move in highlighting the importance of Nursing.

Today Nursing Studies, which is part of the University's School of Health and Social Science, continues educating undergraduates and postgraduates as well as carrying out research to improve the patient experience including looking at healthcare organisation and policy and how individuals and their families experience health and illness. Each year the Department of Nursing Studies also hosts the Elsie Stephenson Memorial Lecture, where delegates meet to discuss key issues affecting their profession.

The Polish School of Medicine (1941–1949)

The University of Edinburgh has a rich history and strong focus on international collaboration, a spirit embodied in the setting up of the Polish School of Medicine during the Second World War. The school closed when the war ended, but the University has retained links with Poland through its alumni and friends, and the school's memorial fund and also hosts the school's historical collection.

The Polish School was established following the German invasion of Poland and the subsequent surrender of France. A large number of Polish armed forces evacuated from occupied France were stationed in Eastern Scotland and the school was opened to support the Polish army doctors and encourage them to meet and work with their British colleagues. It also helped Polish medical students to continue their studies with teaching staff from the pre-war Medical Academies of Krakow, Lwow, Poznan, Warsaw and Wilnow. As Jozef Brodzki wrote in 1942:

> The creation of the Polish Medical Faculty in Scotland is an event unique not only in the history of these two countries, but also in the history of the civilised world. History has never known of any state which set up its own university with its own professors lecturing to its own students in their own native tongue on foreign soil as part of a foreign university.[8]

Most of the teaching at the school – whose first Dean, Professor Antoni Jurasz, had been Professor of Surgery at the Medical Academy

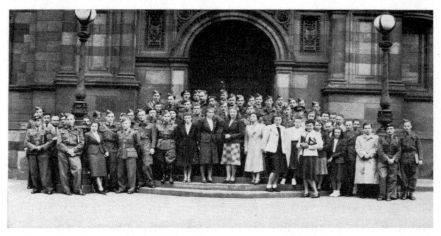

Students from the Polish Medical School, pictured on the steps of McEwan Hall in 1945.

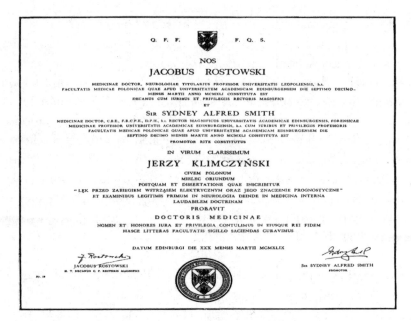

MD diploma from the Polish Medical School, 1949.

of Poznan – was carried out in Polish. A library of Polish textbooks was set up, the British Council helped to run English language courses and the first English–Polish medical dictionary was produced. Polish civilians – some of whom had completed their secondary school education in Britain – were also allowed to matriculate. In total more than 330 students enrolled; 227 – including 46 women – received medical diplomas, while 19 medical degrees were awarded.

The school was also a catalyst in enabling Polish students to study other courses at the University, which included the setting up of a Polish Veterinary Teaching Unit in 1943 at the University's Royal (Dick) School of Veterinary Studies. The example set by Edinburgh influenced other institutions, including Liverpool University, where a Polish School of Architecture was opened in 1942, and Oxford, where a Polish Faculty of Law was set up in 1944.

Although the final examinations for the Polish Medical School took place in 1949, the story does not end there. After the war the graduates and staff retained their links with the University; and since 1966 – the 25th anniversary of the founding of the school – alumni have travelled from across the world to Edinburgh for quinquennial reunions. In 1986 they established a memorial fund to provide scholarships for Polish doctors and medical scientists to undertake research in Edinburgh. The fund also supports the Professor Antoni Jurasz Lectureship, enabling a nominated head of department from Edinburgh Medical School to visit Poland. As a result, links have been built up with medical schools and research institutes across Poland.

To date, the fund has enabled medical scientists and doctors to come to Edinburgh to undertake research, further study or participate in the Medical Teaching Organisation Summer School; medical students and doctors have also come to Edinburgh under the auspices of the Boloz-Kulesza Trust Fund and the Dr James and Bozena Bain Memorial Trust Fund.

Today the University of Edinburgh is developing research and teaching partnerships with Poland, sharing expertise and promoting student mobility at undergraduate and postgraduate levels. In early March 2009, the University signed a memorandum of understanding with Poznan University of Medical Sciences and there are plans to establish a similar agreement with the Collegium Medicum of the Jagiellonian University in Krakow.

Clinical Developments and Research

In addition to advances and proactive initiatives to enhance medical training, the last hundred years has seen enormous strides in research to develop treatments for illnesses and disease. This includes the work of Norman Dott, who started his studies in the same year that the First World War broke out and who would become Britain's first full-time neurosurgeon.[9]

The permanent limp that had been caused by a motorcycle accident meant that Dott was not eligible to fight at the Front. This accident, which had spared him from the bloody battlefields of Belgium and France, caused him to become fascinated with Medicine. The eight weeks spent receiving treatment at the Royal Infirmary of Edinburgh had convinced him – even though he had started working as an apprentice joiner and engineer – that Medicine was his vocation.

After completing his degree, Dott worked as a resident house surgeon at the Royal Infirmary before gaining a clinical tutorship in surgery while also lecturing in Physiology. In 1923 he became assistant surgeon at the Chalmers and Deaconess Hospitals in Edinburgh as well as a fellow of the Royal College of Surgeons of Edinburgh. It was, however, a Rockefeller Travelling Fellowship that enabled him to travel to Boston, USA, to work with the eminent endocrinologist Harvey Cushing – considered the father of modern neurosurgery – that was to shape his future career. Dott returned to Edinburgh with an intense interest in the new medical specialty of 'surgical neurology' and in 1931 was appointed Associate Neurological Surgeon at the Royal Infirmary, subsequently also lecturing in Neurological Surgery at the University. Right at the outset he was to gain international recognition with an operation to contain a ruptured aneurysm in the Circle of Willis, a network of blood vessels at the base of the brain – the first such operation of its kind.

Carrying out this pioneering brain surgery in 1931 was a bold move, not least because the patient, Colin Black, a 53-year-old solicitor, was a governor of the Royal Hospital for Sick Children and Dott, at the age of 33, was relatively unestablished. Black, who was suffering from a headache, neck pain, tingling down his left side and vomiting, was diagnosed as having a brain haemorrhage. Further haemorrhages occurred eight and 14 days later, the last leaving the patient in a coma. Bed rest was the approved treatment for hemorrhages, but even if patients recovered from such incidents, as with Black's case, the bleeding often recurred.

Black's operation, which took three hours and 40 minutes, involved cutting open the skull to expose the ruptured aneurysm, before wrapping and reinforcing it with muscle. Dott estimated the chances of Black's spontaneous recovery as 'very poor indeed, probably not more than 10 per cent'.[10] Dott's brother Eric later recalled how an eminent surgeon had warned Dott against operating, saying that it would not be successful and would damage his career and reputation.[11] Yet the operation was a success and Black lived for another 11 years with no further haemorrhages. Dott's fame spread, but although he carried out two more such operations the same year, he then seemed to abandon the technique. Aneurysm clipping was subsequently introduced in 1937 with clips that had been designed by Cushing as early as 1911.[12] Two years after his operation on Black, Dott gained further recognition when he performed the first angiogram to diagnose an intracranial haemorrhage.

Dott raised funds to establish a Department of Surgical Neurology in the Royal Infirmary, and this, often referred to as Ward 20, was officially opened in 1939. While the department remained at the hospital during the Second World War, the Brain Injuries Unit moved to Bangour – 15 miles west of Edinburgh – for protection from air raids. At the same time Dott was made Consultant in Neurosurgery to the Army in Scotland as well as Consultant Neurosurgeon to the Emergency Medical Service. The unit dealt with about 1,000 cases a year – half of them civilians and half from the armed forces.[13]

In 1960, just two years before his retirement, Dott's grand vision of a purpose-built, fully-comprehensive Department of Surgical Neurology became a reality at the Edinburgh's Western General Hospital. Today his legacy remains; Neurology and Neurosurgery are still based at the Western General Hospital while Neuroscience also flourishes at other University sites within the Centres for Clinical Brain Sciences, Cognitive Neurosystems, Integrative Physiology and most recently the Centre for Neuroregeneration, which incorporates the new Euan MacDonald Centre for Motor Neurone Disease Research.

Brain surgery is not the only surgical discipline in which great strides have been made in Edinburgh. Another surgeon to make his mark in the 20th century was Michael Woodruff, who performed the UK's first successful kidney transplant. The operation, which took place in 1960, also paved the way for Edinburgh to open the first custom-built transplant unit of its kind eight years later.

Born in London, Woodruff spent much of his youth in Australia where he read Electrical Engineering at the University of Melbourne before switching to a degree in Medicine in 1940, gaining the Master of Surgery there in 1941. During the war he joined the Australian Army Medical Corps and, after being captured by the Japanese, was held in

Changi Prison Camp. Amid the horrendous conditions of prison life, he devised a way of extracting juice from grasses to ward off vitamin deficiencies such as beri beri. The concoctions he made were apparently foul-tasting, but did serve to keep those who drank them healthy.

After the war Woodruff returned to Britain, where he became fascinated with overcoming the rejection of transplanted organs by the immune system. He worked as a tutor in surgery at Sheffield University, then as a senior lecturer at the University of Aberdeen, before moving to New Zealand in 1953 as Professor in Surgery at the University in Dunedin. At these posts he continued his research on transplant rejection and began to investigate its prevention using anti-lymphocytic serum with research on laboratory animals, which came to fruition later in his career.

Woodruff was appointed Professor of Surgical Science at Edinburgh in 1957. With no anti-rejection drugs available, during the 1950s several unsuccessful attempts at organ transplantation took place. But in 1954 the first successful kidney transplant was carried out in Boston, USA. This was between 23-year-old identical twins whose matching tissue type eliminated any problems of immune rejection, but it was many years before such operations would be performed between non-identical pairs.

In 1960 Woodruff became the first person in the UK to successfully carry out a kidney transplant. The operation was performed at Leith Hospital. Lewis Abbot, a 49-year-old steel warehouseman, received a kidney from his identical twin brother, Martin. Martin returned to work three weeks later, Lewis after 15 weeks. Both died six years later, although of causes unrelated to kidney disease. The operation caught the imagination of the public so much that a reporter from the *Daily Express*, in a ruse to visit the twins in hospital, persuaded their aunt to pass him off as one of her nephews.[14]

The second kidney transplant in Edinburgh, which took place the following year, between a brother and sister, was not so successful. Woodruff used a large dose of x-radiation to suppress the immune system and thereby reduce the chance of organ rejection. The irradiation, however, had left the patient at high risk of infection. Before the patient was transferred from the Western General Hospital to the Royal Infirmary, Woodruff, who was thought not to have any *Staphylococcus aureus* bacteria on his skin, personally scrubbed and disinfected the ambulance.[15] However, despite these precautions, the patient died 30 days after the operation from septicaemia. No other kidney transplant was carried out in Edinburgh until the first immunosuppressant drug, azathrioprine – deemed safer than irradiation – came into use. It was the second such operation worldwide using this drug and the transplant patient survived for more than 20 years.

During the 1960s Woodruff found that by wiping out an animal's lymphocytes with anti-lymphocyte serum he could prevent immunological rejection and prolong the survival of a transplanted kidney. He and his team worked to understand the immunological mechanisms behind this and made a serum against human lymphocytes in horses with a view to using it in transplant patients. In 1968 the Nuffield Foundation, in recognition of his major contribution to transplant surgery, funded The Nuffield Transplant Surgery Unit at the Western General Hospital, which opened under Woodruff's directorship. Six patients could be treated at once and anti-lymphocyte serum was used routinely in combination with immunosuppressant drugs to prevent organ rejection. Woodruff was made a Fellow of the Royal Society in 1968 and in 1969 he received a knighthood for Services to Medicine.

His pioneering work placed Edinburgh at the forefront of transplant surgery, paving the way for the Scottish Liver Transplant Surgery Unit – one of seven such units in the UK – to be established in 1992 at the Royal Infirmary of Edinburgh. Three years later the Renal Transplant Unit joined it at the hospital. The Scottish Pancreas Transplant Programme was established in 2000. Together these units perform around 180 routine transplants each year, while between 60 and 70 patients with acute liver failure also receive emergency transplants at the Scottish Liver Unit.

It was not only in surgery, however, that medical advances were being made. A revolutionary treatment for tuberculosis (TB) devised in Edinburgh has served to improve the health of millions across the globe. By the end of the Second World War TB was still a major health scourge and Edinburgh was one of the few places in Europe where TB prevalence was increasing. By 1948, TB was claiming a victim every two hours in Scotland and was a major cause of death in young people in the city.

The person to address this was John Crofton, who had graduated from the University of Cambridge in Natural Sciences in 1933 before finishing his clinical training at St Thomas's Hospital in London in 1937. He arrived in Edinburgh in 1951 to take up the post of Professor of Respiratory Diseases and Tuberculosis, having been in charge of early clinical trials of the first anti TB antibiotic, streptomycin, at the Brompton Hospital's Medical Research Council TB unit.

His work in Edinburgh was to herald a revolution in the treatment of TB, with what became known as the 'Edinburgh Method'. On arrival, Crofton was put in charge of the 400 tuberculosis beds across three hospitals in the city, but with around 50,000 TB cases in Britain at that time this was hardly adequate. Edinburgh TB patients faced a year-long wait for a hospital bed. Crofton wasted no time in negotiating more beds and consultant posts to rectify this woeful shortage.

Two new drugs had recently become available for treating TB, para-aminosalicylic acid (PAS) and isoniazid, but no one knew the best way to use them in relation to the older drug streptomycin. Some patients treated with a single agent recovered, others relapsed. Since this treatment failure was attributed to the microbe becoming resistant to the drug, Crofton decided to administer all three drugs together.

The outcome was astonishing – patients were being cured. Between 1954 and 1957 Crofton's team halved the TB notification rates in Edinburgh and he predicted that within 20 years TB would be under firm control in the city. In fact, it took a third of this time, with the disease almost eliminated within six years. Not only had Crofton found a way of treating this potentially fatal illness, he also realised that if the medication was taken appropriately patients did not need to stay in hospital, enabling beds to be freed up for those with other respiratory diseases. He presented his results at the British Medical Association's annual meeting in 1958 and published them in the *British Medical*

Journal in 1959. This paper boldly began, 'The right use of modern methods of chemotherapy now makes it possible to aim at 100 per cent success in the treatment of pulmonary tuberculosis.' [16]

But Crofton's results were greeted with scepticism. To counteract such disbelief, he initiated a multi-centre clinical trial of the Edinburgh Method involving 23 countries, with what was possibly the first international collaborative trial for disease therapy. The outcome of this trial meant that the success of the Edinburgh Method could no longer be contested and it was adopted across Europe and North America.

Crofton, a man of immense energy, did not to stop there. In addition to continuing his research he held many roles, including that of Dean of the Faculty of Medicine, 1963-1966, Vice-Principal of the University of Edinburgh between 1969 and 1971 and President of the Royal College of Physicians of Edinburgh from 1973 to 1976. He co-edited a classic textbook, *Respiratory Medicine*, now in its fifth edition, and was knighted in 1977.

Crofton, a father of five, was also a campaigner, and in later life he sought to improve public health more generally. In the 1970s with his wife Eileen, he helped to found Action on Smoking and Health (ASH) through which they successfully lobbied for anti-smoking legislation – Scotland was the first place in Britain to introduce a smoking ban in public places. He also led the Alcohol Forum, set up by the Department of Health with drink companies, and in 1998 he helped found TB Alert, a charity supporting TB projects around the world and promoting awareness of the disease.

Even after he retired in 1977 Crofton continued to work tirelessly for the causes in which he so passionately believed. He was the first chairman of the Tobacco and Health Committee of the International Union against Tuberculosis and Lung Disease, and acted as an advisor to the World Health Organisation on TB, which included visits to Nepal to advise on TB treatment there. His impact was such that following his death in 2009 a motion in the Scottish Parliament stated: 'The Parliament is united in sadness at the death of Sir John Crofton and considers that Scotland has lost one of its most inspirational health pioneers.'[17] In honour of this outstanding Edinburgh clinical academic, the University named the Chair of Respiratory Medicine after Sir John Crofton in 2010, the first incumbent being Professor Chris Haslett, also the inaugural Director of the University's Queen's Medical Research Institute.

New treatments for medical conditions were not the only way in which countless lives were being saved and by the 1960s the use of vaccines to prevent infections was having a strong impact reducing the spread of infections. One such infection was the potentially fatal 'serum hepatitis' caused by hepatitis B virus. The work of Kenneth Murray, alongside that of his wife Noreen, on the development of recombinant DNA technology in Edinburgh was to lead to the first synthetic vaccine against this highly contagious, blood-borne virus. Despite the millions that could have been earned from the royalties of the patent, Murray instead put the money into a charitable foundation – the Darwin Trust of Edinburgh – which supports educational and research activities.

Although Murray left school at the age of 16, when he became a laboratory technician at Boots the Chemist in Nottingham, and later at Glaxo's streptomycin plant at Ulverston, he carried on studying part-time and eventually gained a first class degree in chemistry and then a PhD in microbiology from the University of Birmingham. He arrived in Edinburgh in 1967 after a period of postdoctoral research in Protein Chemistry at Stanford University. At the time Edinburgh was the only university in the UK to have a department of Molecular Biology and Murray, who was among the leaders in developing DNA sequencing, and his wife Noreen, a distinguished molecular geneticist, worked there until their retirement.

In the 1960s genetic engineering was viewed as an obscure discipline and was often treated with scepticism. Despite this Murray forged ahead and pioneered the use of bacterial enzymes to cut strands of DNA at specific points for cloning or isolating individual genes. Today genetic engineering is fully integrated into medical research – not least with the sequencing of the human genome – but as Murray himself recalled in a newspaper interview: 'A number of people laughed at us and said it was all daydream and just pie in the sky.'[18]

However he was to prove the sceptics wrong and his blue-skies thinking paid off. In 1978 he joined some of the world's leading genetic engineers to form a company called Biogen to exploit this new technology. He then set about cloning parts of the human hepatitis B virus with a view to making a synthetic vaccine.

The first hurdle was to find live hepatitis B virus. Fortunately Murray was able to gain access to blood samples that had been taken during a tragic hepatitis outbreak at the Edinburgh Transplant Unit in 1969–70 and used in research on the serology of hepatitis B in the Department of Medical Microbiology. The outbreak started after a chronic renal patient was transfused with infected blood, leading to dozens of staff and patients becoming infected and 11 deaths.

Work began in June 1978. Because of the fear of genetic engineering and the highly contagious nature of the material, much of it had to be carried out in the Category Four containment laboratory at Porton Down, Wiltshire, the UK Government's germ warfare establishment. Despite this, by November of the same year the scientists had succeeded in making the hepatitis B protein they needed. This laid the foundations for both a diagnostic test for hepatitis B infection and the development of a synthetic vaccine. By Christmas they had applied for the first patents.

The production of a vaccine is a long process, but by 1984 safety trials in chimpanzees were completed and the world's first synthetic vaccine was ready for use in humans. It proved to be not only effective, but both safer and cheaper than earlier vaccines derived from blood products. Today the global hepatitis B vaccine market exceeds $1 billion annually and is expected to continue to grow as more countries adopt World Health Organisation recommendations for the vaccinations of newborns, teenagers, healthcare workers and other groups at risk of infection.

Murray's philanthropic act in setting up the Darwin Trust of Edinburgh to channel the millions he could have received from royalties into good causes has earned him the title of the 'Robin Hood' of medical research. 'I could have taken the money but I don't need to, I don't particularly want a Rolls-Royce,' said Murray, who was knighted in 1993. 'It has been a fairy story I suppose. I have actually got a lot of satisfaction out of the Trust.'[19] Murray was appointed as a Fellow to the Royal Society in 1979, with Noreen becoming a fellow in 1982.

In addition to finding new treatments or preventing disease, Edinburgh academics have also played an influential role in informing and shaping healthcare policies. One such is academic Sir Patrick Forrest, whose appointment as Regius Professor of Clinical Surgery in 1971 helped establish Edinburgh as one of the leading international centres in breast disease research and treatment. Forrest was instrumental in setting up a national breast screening programme in Britain, an initiative that has ensured much earlier diagnosis of breast cancer and as a result better disease outcomes.

Born in Lanarkshire, Forrest graduated from St Andrews in 1945, before spending two years as a Surgeon Lieutenant in the Royal Naval Volunteer Reserve. He was later to work as a senior lecturer at the Western Infirmary's Department of Surgery in Glasgow and gained a Masters of Surgery with Honours and a Gold Medal for his early experimental research into the pathophysiology of peptic ulceration. He received a Doctorate of Medicine with similar distinction for his work on pituitary ablation in the treatment of advanced breast cancer and, when he became Professor of Surgery at the Welsh National School of Medicine in 1962, he continued studying gastric physiology and breast disease and set up research laboratories.

After arriving in Edinburgh he initiated an extensive research programme which ranged from looking at the endocrinology of tumours to the screening of healthy women. In 1981, he also took up a position as Chief Scientist and four years later he was appointed by the then Minister of Health, Kenneth Clarke, to chair a committee to report on breast cancer screening. Britain's death rate from breast cancer was then one of the highest in Western Europe. Early diagnosis of the disease, which is more common in older women, has been crucial in improving survival rates. The Forrest report recommended that women between the ages of 50 and 64 be screened every three years. In 1988 the first women were invited to take part in the National Breast Cancer Screening Programme; when the initiative was first introduced it detected more than 16,000 cases a year.

Today almost two out of three women with breast cancer survive their disease beyond 20 years, with early diagnosis no doubt having a significant impact along with improved treatments. Forrest, who was Regius Chair of Clinical Surgery until 1988, was also particularly interested in hormonal manipulation of breast cancer and was the main driving force behind the development of the successful multi-centre UK breast cancer treatment trials that started in the 1970s. In 1986 he was knighted for his Services to Surgery.

Prion Disease Surveillance in Edinburgh

In 1990 the UK surveillance unit for Creutzfeldt-Jakob Disease (CJD) was established at the University of Edinburgh. The centre was set up in response to concerns that bovine spongiform encephalopathy (BSE) might spread to humans through the consumption of contaminated beef. The unit is spearheaded by professors Bob Will and James Ironside, who with other staff members have played a key role in influencing Government policy to limit the spread of variant CJD, particularly by membership of the Spongiform Encephalopathy Advisory Committee.

The first case of BSE – referred to in the headlines as 'mad cow disease' – was identified in the UK in 1986. Like CJD, it belongs to the class of diseases known as transmissible spongiform encephalopathies (TSEs) that are caused by infectious proteins called prions and cause fatal degeneration of the central nervous system. It subsequently transpired that BSE was spread to cattle in their feed, which contained prions from sheep infected with scrapie – also a TSE. As thousands of cases of BSE were identified, the experts and public alike feared that humans who ate contaminated beef might then develop a form of CJD.

The unit was given the task of monitoring CJD cases throughout the UK and Europe and in 1996 they published a paper in *The Lancet,* alarmingly entitled 'A New Variant of Creutzfeld-Jakob Disease in the UK'.[20] This reported four deaths from a distinctive form of CJD which affected young people in particular. Later research showed that this variant CJD was caused by an abnormal prion protein with identical characteristics to the BSE agent, indicating that it had entered the food chain and had spread to humans.

The surveillance unit also carries out extensive research into the pathology of the disease and aims to improve diagnosis, which at present can only be confirmed by post-mortem examination. In 2004 researchers at the unit identified blood transfusion as an additional mode of the spread of variant CJD.[21] This startling finding led the UK Government to ban blood donation by anybody who had previously had a blood transfusion in case they had received blood from an infected donor. The CJD unit followed up their observation by examining 12,674 random appendix and tonsils samples for signs of the abnormal prion protein. They calculated that around 4,000 people in the UK could be carriers and potentially develop or pass on the disease.

There have been more than 160 deaths from variant CJD since 1995 but, following the peak of 28 deaths in 2000, incidence has declined with just three cases reported in 2009. However, the long incubation period could mean that some people are still incubating the disease and the surveillance unit remains pivotal in fully understanding its impact.

Dolly the Sheep (1996–2003)

On 22 February 1997 another major breakthrough in Edinburgh made headlines across the world. It was announced that a sheep named Dolly had become the first mammal to be cloned from the DNA of an adult cell. The research, carried out by Ian Wilmut and colleagues at The Roslin Institute, sparked controversy and ethical debates over cell cloning. It also heralded huge new opportunities in the field of stem cell research for the study of human diseases. Dolly's birth was described in a paper entitled 'Viable Offspring Derived from Fetal and Adult Mammalian Cells' in the journal *Nature*, and was proclaimed by *Science* magazine as the breakthrough of the year.[22] It showed that adult somatic cells were much more flexible than previously thought, paving the way for stem cell research to help model disease in a culture dish with implications for both drug development and potential stem cell therapies.

Wilmut initially chose to study Agriculture at Nottingham University but developed an increasing interest in research. After spending the summer of 1966 working in a research laboratory in Cambridge, he decided to remain there for his PhD following which he moved to

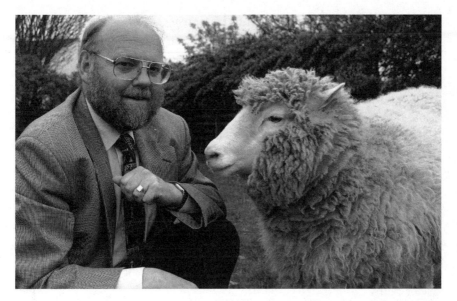

Ian Wilmut and Dolly, the cloned sheep.

Scotland, to a post at the Animal Breeding and Research Organisation just outside Edinburgh, which later became The Roslin Institute and joined with the University of Edinburgh in 2008.

The arrival of Dolly caused a tremendous stir as journalists congregated at The Roslin Institute near the small, sleepy village of Roslin in Midlothian. With a tongue-in-cheek sense of humour, scientists named the lamb Dolly after a very different kind of celebrity – the busty country and western singer Dolly Parton. This was because when cloning Dolly they had taken DNA from the mammary gland of a six-year-old sheep. They then fused this with a ewe's unfertilised egg from which DNA had been removed in a process known as somatic cell nuclear transfer. Once the cloned embryo had reached a suitable age in tissue culture it was transferred to a surrogate mother sheep, which later gave birth to the cloned lamb.

Although Dolly's birth was announced to the public in February 1997, she had entered the world more than seven months earlier. Her birth was kept quiet at first so that scientists could prepare their results for publication before announcing her arrival. Dolly, a Finn Dorset sheep, was the only success out of nearly 300 cloning attempts. Of 300 eggs, only 29 had grown enough to be transferred into surrogate sheep. While 13 sheep became pregnant, only one ewe delivered a healthy lamb – Dolly. Her birth proved that genetic material from a specialised adult cell, such as an udder cell, could be reprogrammed to generate an entire new organism. Prior to this, scientists had believed that once adult cells became specialised – for instance to create liver cells – they had been permanently changed. So the birth of Dolly opened up whole new avenues for the field of stem cell research.

Despite being in the media spotlight, Dolly lived a quiet life at The Roslin Institute. She bred with a Welsh mountain ram, producing lambs Bonnie; Sally and Rosy (twins) and Lucy, Darcy and Cotton (triplets). She developed arthritis and a progressive lung disease, and at the age of six she was put down. A post-mortem examination revealed a lung cancer which is common in sheep and was not thought to be the result of her being cloned.

Dolly's legacy lives on. She was conserved by taxidermists and visitors can see her at the National Museum of Scotland in Edinburgh. In promoting public understanding of science, she has travelled since death to open a new science museum in Budapest. More importantly, scientists have taken forward the breakthrough of her birth and are investigating the use of stem cells to treat a range of disease including Parkinson's Disease, multiple sclerosis and motor neurone disease. Wilmut became the Director of the University's Medical Research Council Centre for Regenerative Medicine in 2005, where this work is progressing. He became a fellow of the Royal Society in 2002 and was knighted in the 2008 New Year Honours.

Where to Now?
The dawning of the millennium heralded a new era for medicine in Edinburgh. After being based in the grand, Italian-renaissance style building at Teviot Place for 118 years, the University of Edinburgh Medical School moved to Little France, an area so-named because Mary Queen of Scots' entourage set up camp there while she was in residence at the nearby Craigmillar Castle in the 1560s. This saw a new teaching building – the Chancellor's Building – open in 2002, next door to the

new Royal Infirmary of Edinburgh. The hospital was officially opened in 2003 after 124 years at Lauriston Place. As well as bringing teaching and medical practice alongside, there was a further vision – to ensure that medical research was fully integrated among these disciplines. In 2005 the £50 million Queen's Medical Research Institute was opened beside the Chancellor's Building. More than 600 researchers are based at the Institute within three centres – the Centres for Reproductive Biology, Inflammation Research and Cardiovascular Science. As well as a strong focus on translational medicine – taking research from the laboratory bench to improve treatment of the patient – researchers are encouraged to work collaboratively across different disciplines. With the scientists also based at the Chancellor's Building, there are more than 1,000 researchers on the Little France site.

A state of the art Clinical Research Imaging Centre was also opened in the lower levels of the Queen's Medical Research Insitute in 2010, as part of a collaboration with NHS Lothian. The centre houses a computerised assisted tomography (CT) scanner, which can take 3D images of the heart within a single heartbeat, an MRI scanner for research and a PET scanner for clinical diagnosis.

Groundbreaking research by members of the University's Medical School is also carried out at other sites across the city, including the Western General Hospital, where researchers from the Medical Research Council Human Genetics Unit and Cancer Research UK have come together to form the Institute of Genetics and Molecular Medicine.

In the meantime major developments at Little France are ongoing. Plans for the area include creating one of the top 10 centres for Biomedical Research and Development in Europe with an initiative known as Edinburgh BioQuarter. The project, a partnership between the University, NHS Lothian and Scottish Enterprise, involves developing a Life Sciences Park behind the Royal Infirmary. The first flagship building on the BioQuarter will be the Scottish Centre for Regenerative Medicine, relocating the centre's scientists from the Chancellor's Building while other developments include a £60 million building for scientists from The Roslin Insitue and a new £40 million teaching building for the Royal (Dick) School of Veterinary Studies at the Easter Bush campus.

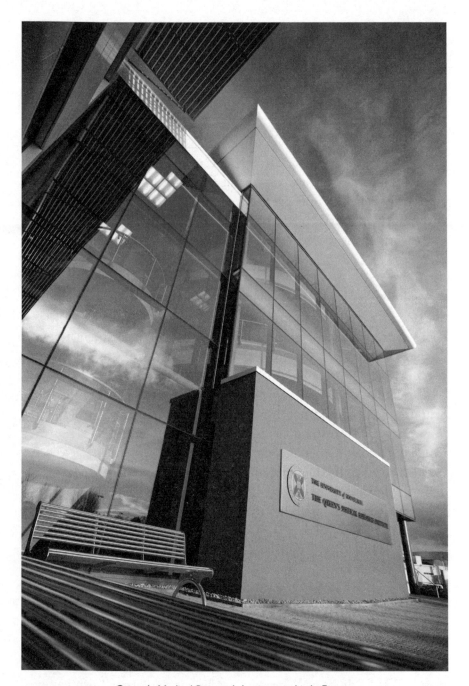

Queen's Medical Research Institute at Little France.

A £10 million donation from the children's author JK Rowling is also enabling the setting up of the Anne Rowling Regenerative Neurology Clinic. This will place patients at the heart of research to improve outcomes for multiple sclerosis and other neurodegenerative diseases with patient-based studies to help find treatments that could slow disease progression, with the eventual aim of stopping and reversing it.

All this is clear evidence of the continuing emphasis placed by the University of Edinburgh on training the next generation of doctors and researchers. As scientific knowledge continues apace, we are learning more and more about the human body. The more we learn the more there is to understand. And, as history has often told us, sometimes what is least expected is the most astounding.

Endnotes

CHAPTER I

1 Anderson, RD, Lynch, M, Phillipson, N. *The University of Edinburgh: An Illustrated History*. Edinburgh University Press, 2003.

2 Boerhaave, H. *Atrocis, nec descripti prius, morbis historia: Secundum medicae artis leges conscripta*. Lugduni Batavorum; Ex officine Boutestenian, 1724.

3 Fraser, A. *The Building of Old College: Adam, Playfair and the University of Edinburgh*. Edinburgh University Press, 1989.

4 Craig, WS. *History of the Royal College of Physicians, Edinburgh*. Blackwell, 1976.

5 Lobban, RD. *Edinburgh and the Medical Revolution*. Cambridge University Press, 1980.

6 Craig WS. *History of the Royal College of Physicians, Edinburgh*. Blackwell, 1976.

7 Quoted from Robert Sibbald's autobiography at http://www.rcpe.ac.uk/library/read/college/physic-garden/physic-garden.php

8 Blackdan, S. *A Tradition of Excellence: A Brief History of Medicine in Edinburgh*. Duncan Flockhart, 1981.

9 Kaufman, M. *Medical Teaching in Edinburgh During the 18th and 19th Centuries*. The Royal College of Surgeons of Edinburgh, 2003.

10 Ibid.

11 Fyffe, WJ. 'Reminiscences of an Army-Surgeon'. Collection of Pamphlets vol. 9, Contemporary Medical Archives Centre, RAMC 423, 1889

12 Fraser, AG. *The Building of Old College: Adam, Playfair and the University of Edinburgh*. Edinburgh University Press, 1989.

13 Rosner, L. *Medical Education in the Age of Improvement: Edinburgh Students and Apprentices 1760–1826*. Edinburgh University Press. 1991.

14 Lobban, RD. *Edinburgh and the Medical Revolution*. Cambridge University Press, 1980.

15 Monro, A (secundus). *Observations on the Structure and Functions of the Nervous System*. William Creech, 1783.

16 Dow, DA (ed). *The Influence of Scottish Medicine: An Historical Assessment of its International Impact*. Parthenon Publishing Group, 1988.

17 Lobban, RD. *Edinburgh and the Medical Revolution*. Cambridge University Press, 1980.

18 Darwin, D. *The Correspondence of Charles Darwin 1821–1836*. Cambridge University Press, 1985.

19 Kaufman, M. *Medical Teaching in Edinburgh During the 18th and 19th Centuries*. The Royal College of Surgeons of Edinburgh, 2003.

20 Lobban, RD. *Edinburgh and the Medical Revolution*. Cambridge University Press, 1980.

21 Fraser, A. *The Building of Old College: Adam, Playfair and the University of Edinburgh*. Edinburgh University Press, 1989.

22 Kaufman, M. *Medical Teaching in Edinburgh During the 18th and 19th Centuries*. The Royal College of Surgeons of Edinburgh, 2003.

23 Ibid.

24 Ibid.

25 A scrap book compiled by Monro tertius, University of Edinburgh Library.

CHAPTER 2

1 Oriel, JD. 'Eminent Venereologists – Benjamin Bell', *Genitourinary Medicine*, 65(5), 1989.

2 Macintyre, I and MacLaren, I (eds). *Surgeons' Lives – Royal College of Surgeons of Edinburgh: An Anthology of College Fellows over 500 Years*. Royal College of Surgeons, 2005.

3 Ibid.

4 *Gazeteer of Scotland: James Syme*. http://www.geo.ed.ac.uk/scotgaz/people/famousfirst988.html.

5 Gordon, R. *Great Medical Disasters*. Stein and Day, 1983.

6 Macintyre, I and MacLaren, I (eds). *Surgeons' Lives – Royal College of Surgeons of Edinburgh: An Anthology of College Fellows over 500 Years*. Royal College of Surgeons, 2005.

7 Heath, C. *Injuries and diseases of the jaws*. John Churchill & Sons, 1868.

8 Shepherd, JA. *Simpson and Syme of Edinburgh*. E&S Livingstone, 1969.

9 Ibid.

10 Ibid.

11 Walker, K. *Joseph Lister*. Hutchison, 1956.

12 Shepherd, JA. *Simpson and Syme of Edinburgh*. E&S Livingstone, 1969.

13 Ibid.

14 Simpson, M. *Simpson the Obstetrician*. Victor Gollancz, 1972.

15 Ibid.

16 Ibid.

17 Ibid.

18 Ibid.

19 Ibid.

20 Duns, J. *Memoir of Sir James Y Simpson*. Edmonston and Douglas, 1873.

21 Simpson, M. *Simpson the Obstetrician*. Victor Gollancz, 1972.

22 Ibid.

23 Drife, J. 'The Start of Life: a History of Obstetrics', *Postgraduate Medical Journal*, 78, 2002. Available from: http://pmj.bmj.com/cgi/content/full/78/919/311.

24 Simpson, M. *Simpson the Obstetrician*. Victor Gollancz, 1972.

25 Drife, J. 'The Start of Life: A History of Obstetrics', *Postgraduate Medical Journal*, 78, 2002. Available from: http://pmj.bmj.com/cgi/contentfull/78/919/311.

26 Simpson, M. *Simpson the Obstetrician*. Victor Gollancz, 1972.
27 Ibid.
28 Atkinson, RS. *James Simpson and Chloroform*. Priory Press, 1973.
29 Ibid.
30 Walker, K. *Joseph Lister*. Hutchison, 1956.
31 Ibid.
32 Ibid.
33 Ibid.
34 Ibid.
35 Ibid.
36 Guthrie, D. *Lord Lister*. E&S Livingstone, 1949.
37 Walker, K. *Joseph Lister*. Hutchison, 1956.
38 Guthrie, D. *Lord Lister*. E&S Livingstone, 1949.
39 Walker, K. *Joseph Lister*. Hutchison, 1956.
40 Ibid.
41 Guthrie, D. *Lord Lister*. E&S Livingstone, 1949.
42 Cameron, H. *Joseph Lister: The Friend of Man*. Heinemann, 1948.
43 Walker, K. *Joseph Lister*. Hutchison, 1956.
44 Ibid.
45 Cameron, H. *Joseph Lister: The Friend of Man*. Heinemann, 1948.
46 Walker, K. *Joseph Lister*. Hutchison, 1956.
47 Guthrie, D. *Lord Lister*. E&S Livingstone, 1949.
48 Cartwright, F. *Joseph Lister: The Man Who Made Surgery Safe*. Weidenfeld and Nicolson, 1963.
49 Cameron, H. *Joseph Lister: The Friend of Man*. Heinemann, 1948.
50 Godlee, R. *Lord Lister*. Macmillan, 1918.

CHAPTER 3
1 Scott, S and Duncan, C. *Return of the Black Death*. Wiley, 2004.
2 Tait, HP. *A Doctor and Two Policemen: A History of Edinburgh Health Department 1862–1974*. EDC Environmental Health Department, 1974.
3 Scott, S and Duncan, C. *Return of the Black Death*. Wiley, 2004.
4 Ibid.
5 Tait, HP. *A Doctor and Two Policemen: A History of Edinburgh Health Department 1862–1974*. EDC Environmental Health Department, 1974.
6 Bhopal, R and Last, J. *Public Health: Past, Present and Future*. The Nuffield Trust, 2004.
7 Brotherston, JHF. *Observations on the Early Public Health Movement in Scotland*. London School of Hygiene and Tropical Medicine Memoir 8. HK Lewis, 1952.
8 Tait, HP. *A Doctor and Two Policemen: A History of Edinburgh Health Department 1862–1974*. EDC Environmental Health Department, 1974.
9 Brotherston, JHF. *Observations on the Early Public Health Movement in*

Scotland. London School of Hygiene and Tropical Medicine Memoir 8. HK Lewis, 1952.

10 Tait, HP. *A Doctor and Two Policemen: A History of Edinburgh Health Department 1862–1974*. EDC Environmental Health Department, 1974.

11 Ibid.

12 Water quality and flooding. www.edinburgh.gov.uk.

13 Brotherston, JHF. *Observations on the Early Public Health Movement in Scotland*. London School of Hygiene and Tropical Medicine Memoir 8. HK Lewis, 1952.

14 Stark, J. *Inquiry into Some Points of the Sanitary State of Edinburgh*. Stark and Co, 1847.

15 Smith, PJ. 'The Foul Burns of Edinburgh: Health Attitudes and Environmental Change', *Scottish Geographical Magazine*, 91, 1975.

16 Ibid.

17 Brotherston, JHF. *Observations on the Early Public Health Movement in Scotland*. London School of Hygiene and Tropical Medicine Memoir 8. HK Lewis, 1952.

18 Alison, WP. *Observations on the Management of the Poor in Scotland and its Effect on Health in the Great Towns*. Blackwood, 1840.

19 Brotherston, JHF. *Observations on the Early Public Health Movement in Scotland*. London School of Hygiene and Tropical Medicine Memoir 8. HK Lewis, 1952.

20 Ibid.

21 Smith, PJ. 'The Foul Burns of Edinburgh: Health Attitudes and Environmental Change', *Scottish Geographical Magazine*, 91, 1975.

22 Tait, HP. *A Doctor and Two Policemen: A History of Edinburgh Health Department 1862–1974*. EDC Environmental Health Department, 1974.

23 Ibid.

24 Ibid.

25 Ibid.

26 Ibid.

27 Ibid.

28 Ibid.

29 Wallace, AT. *Sir Robert Philip: A Pioneer in the Campaign Against Tuberculosis. Medical History* 5(1), 1961.

30 Ibid.

31 Tait, HP. *A Doctor and Two Policemen: A History of Edinburgh Health Department 1862–1974*. EDC Environmental Health Department, 1974.

32 Ibid.

33 Bhopal, R and Last, J. *Public Health: Past, Present and Future*, The Nuffield Trust, 2004.

34 Tait, HP. *A Doctor and Two Policemen: A History of Edinburgh Health Department 1862–1974*. EDC Environmental Health Department, 1974.

CHAPTER 4

1   Savona-Ventura, C. 'Dr James Barry: An Enigmatic Army Medical Doctor',
     Maltese Medical Journal 8(1), 1996.
2   Ibid.
3   Rae, I. *The Strange Story of Dr James Barry*. Longmans, Green and Co,
     1958.
4   Du Preez, HM. 'Dr James Barry: The Early Years Revealed. *South African
     Medical Journal* 98, 2008.
5   Rae, I. *The Strange Story of Dr James Barry*. Longmans, Green and Co,
     1958.
6   Lesson, J and Gray, J. *Women and Medicine*. Tavistock Publications, 1978.
7   Ibid.
8   Roberts, S. *Sophia Jex-Blake: A Woman Pioneer in Ninteenth-Century
     Medical Reform*. Routledge, 1993.
9   Ibid.
10   Ibid.
11   Ibid.
12   Ibid.
13   Ibid.
14   Ibid.
15   Ibid.
16   Ibid.
17   Ibid.
18   Ibid.
19   Ibid.
20   Ibid.
21   Ibid.
22   Ibid.
23   Leneman, L. *Elsie Inglis: Founder of Battlefield Hospitals Run Entirely by
     Women*. NMS Publishing, 1998.
24   Ibid.
25   Ibid.
26   Ibid.

CHAPTER 5

1   Playfair, J. 'Biographical account of the late Dr James Hutton FRS Edin',
     Transactions of the Royal Society of Edinburgh, V, 1805. Reprinted by the
     RSE Scotland Foundation, 1997.
2   McIntyre, DB and McKirdy, A. *James Hutton: The Founder of Modern
     Geology*. The Stationary Office, 1997.
3   Jones, J. *James Hutton: Founder of Modern Geology*. Scotland's Cultural
     Heritage, 1984.
4   Jones, J. *James Hutton: Founder of Modern Geology*. Scotland's Cultural

Heritage, 1984.

5   McIntyre, DB and McKirdy, A. *James Hutton: The Founder of Modern Geology*. The Stationary Office, 1997.

6   Ibid.

7   Playfair, J. *Illustrations of the Huttonian Theory of the Earth*. William Creech, 1802.

8   Pearson, PN. *Nature* 425, 2003.

9   Ferguson, A. *Minutes of the Life and Character of Joseph Black*, MD. Transactions of the Royal Society of Edinburgh, v, 1805. Reprinted by the RSE Scotland Foundation, 1997.

10 Ibid.

11 Ibid.

12 Ibid.

13 Ibid.

14 Eldredge, N. 'The Art of Medicine: What Darwin Learned in Medical School'. *The Lancet* 373, 2009.

15 Barlow, N. *The Autobiography of Charles Darwin*. Collins, 1958.

16 Ibid.

17 Ibid.

18 Ibid.

19 Ibid.

20 Ibid.

21 Desmond, A and Moore, JA. *Darwin's Sacred Cause: How Slavery Shaped Darwin's View of Human Evolution*. Allen Lane, 2009.

22 Barlow, N (ed). *The Autobiography of Charles Darwin*. Collins, 1958.

23 Ibid.

24 Darwin, C. *On the Origin of Species*. John Murray, 1859.

25 Lycett, A. *Conan Doyle: The Man Who Created Sherlock Holmes*. Phoenix, 2007.

26 Ibid.

27 Ibid.

28 Ibid.

29 Conan Doyle, A. 'Gelseminum as a Poison', *British Medical Journal* 2, 1879; reprinted in *BMJ* 339, 2009.

30 Lycett, A. *Conan Doyle: The Man Who Created Sherlock Holmes*. Phoenix, 2007.

31 Ibid.

32 Ibid.

33 Barnes, J. *Arthur and George*. Abbey Books, 2005.

CHAPTER 6

1   Macintyre, I and MacLaren, I (eds). *Surgeons' Lives – Royal College of Surgeons of Edinburgh: An Anthology of College Fellows over 500 Years*.

Royal College of Surgeons, 2005.

2 Charles Bell. Available at http://www.electricscotland.com/history/other/
   bellcharles.htm.

3 Macintyre, I and MacLaren, I (eds). *Surgeons' Lives – Royal College of
   Surgeons of Edinburgh: An Anthology of College Fellows over 500 Years*.
   Royal College of Surgeons, 2005.

4 Loudon, ISL. 'Sir Charles Bell and the Anatomy of Expression', *British
   Medical Journal*, 285, 1982.

5 Hale-White, W. *Great Doctors of the Nineteenth Century*, Edward Arnold,
   1935.

6 Hurt, Z et al. *Great Ideas in the History of Surgery*, Norman Publishing,
   1993.

7 Hale-White, W. *Great Doctors of the Nineteenth Century*,.Edward Arnold,
   1935.

8 De Puy, WH. *Encyclopaedia Britannica: A Dictionary of Arts, Sciences, and
   General Literature*, vol. 3, Peale, 1891.

9 Berry, D. 'Richard Bright (1789–1858): Student Days in Edinburgh',
   Proceedings of the Royal College of Physicians of Edinburgh, 24, 1994.

10 Hale-White, W. *Great Doctors of the Nineteenth Century*, Edward Arnold,
   1935.

11 Graner, JL. 'Addison, Pernicious Anemia and Adrenal Insufficiency',
   Canadian Medical Association, 133, 1985.

12 Highley, S. *On the Constitutional and Local Effects of Disease of the Supra-
   renal Capsules*. Thomas Addison, 1855.

13 Ibid.

14 Hale-White, W. *Great Doctors of the Nineteenth Century*, Edward Arnold,
   1935.

15 Geller, SA. Letter to the editor, *Journal of Genetic Counselling*, 11(5), 2002.

16 Burnby, JGL. 'A Study of the English Apothecary from 1660 to 1760',
   Medical History Supplement 3, 1983

17 Kass, AM and Kass EH. *Perfecting the World: The Life and Times of Dr
   Thomas Hodgkin 1798–1866*. Harcourt Brace Jovanovich, 1998.

18 Ibid.

19 Ibid.

20 Ibid.

21 Ibid.

22 Ibid.

23 *The British Medical Journal*, vol. 2 (no. 771), 1875.

24 Ibid.

25 Jacyna, S. 'John Hughes Bennett and the Discovery of Leukaemia:
   Microscopy in Edinburgh', *Lilliputian Wonders; Papers from a Symposium
   held in the Royal College of Physicians of Edinburgh*, 1995.

26 Bennett, JH. 'Histology, and Use of the Microscope', *Lancet*, 45 (1132),

1845.

27 Syme, J. 'Introductory Lecture to a Course of Clinical Surgery'. *The Lancet*, 2: 526 in Jacyna, S. 'John Hughes Bennett and the Discovery of Leukaemia: Microscopy in Edinburgh', *Lilliputian Wonders; Papers from a Symposium held in the Royal College of Physicians of Edinburgh*, 1995.

28 Bennett, JH. 'Case of Hypertrophy of the Spleen and Liver in which Death Took Place from Suppuration of the Blood', *Edinburgh Medical and Surgical Journal*, 64, 1845.

29 Pillar, GJ. 'Leukaemia: A Brief Historical Review From Ancient Times to 1950', *British Journal of Haematology*, 112, 2001.

30 Warner, JH. 'John Hughes Bennett and the Discovery of Leukaemia – Bennett and the Bloodletting Controversy', *Lilliputian Wonders; papers from a Symposium held in the Royal College of Physicians of Edinburgh*, 1995.

31 Ibid.

32 Parapia, AL. 'History of Bloodletting by Phlebotomy', *British Journal of Haematology*, 143, 1995.

33 Warner, JH 'John Hughes Bennett and the Discovery of Leukaemia – Bennett and the Bloodletting Controversy'. *Papers from a Symposium held in the Royal College of Physicians of Edinburgh*, 1995.

34 Ibid.

35 Kerridge IH, Lowe M; 'Bloodletting: The Story of a Therapeutic Technique', *Medical Journal of Australia* 163, 1995, in DePalma *et al.*, 'Bloodletting: Past and Present', *Journal American College of Surgeons*, 205(1), 2007.

36 Osler, W. *The Principles and Practice of Medicine*. Appleton, 1892.

37 Comrie, JD. *History of Scottish Medicine*, vol. 2, Baillerie, Tyndal and Cox, 1932.

38 Department of Oncology, University of Edinburgh: *History of John Hughes Bennett*. Available at http:www.onc.ed.ac.uk/jhbl/history.htm.

CHAPTER 7

1 Scott, R. 'Edinburgh University General Practice Teaching Unit', *Journal of Medical Education*, vol. 31 no. 9, September 1956.

2 Anon. 'Nursing Teaching Unit's New Name', *Edinburgh Evening News*, 22 January, 1957.

3 Runciman, PJ. Second Elsie Stephenson Memorial Lecture on the occasion of the 25th anniversary of Nursing Studies in the University of Edinburgh. 'Past Aspirations – Present Hopes'. University of Edinburgh, Department of Nursing Studies, 1981.

4 Anon. 'Director, Nursing Teaching Unit, University of Edinburgh', *Nursing Times*, 20 April 1956.

5 Anon. 'Gosh – The Nurse has got an MA!', *The Sunday Post*, 8 May 1960.

6 Anon. 'Nurses in "Queue" for University Course'. *Evening Dispatch*, October 1960.

7   Powell, MB. *Nursing Mirror and Midwives Journal*, 10 March 1967.
8   Dlugolecka-Graham, M. *Polish School of Medicine Historical Collection Project*, The Polish School of Medicine and Historical Collection at the University of Edinburgh, 2004.
9   Todd, NV, Howie, JE, Miller, JD. 'Norman Dott's Contribution to Aneurysm Surgery'. *Journal of Neurology, Neurosurgery and Psychiatry* 53, 1990.
10 Ibid.
11 Rush, C and Shaw, JF. *With Sharp Compassion*. Aberdeen University Press, 1990.
12 Dandy, WE. 'Intracranial Aneurysm of the Internal Carotid Artery: Cured by Operation', *Annals of Surgery* 107, 1938.
13 Rush, C and Shaw, JF. *With Sharp Compassion*. Aberdeen University Press, 1990.
14 Renal Unit of the Royal Infirmary of Edinburgh: History of Kidney Transplantation in Edinburgh. Available from http://renux.dmed.ed.ac.uk/EdREN/Unitbits/historyweb/transplant.htm.
15 Ibid.
16 Crofton, J. 'Chemotherapy of Pulmonary Tuberculosis', *British Medical Journal*, 1(5138), 1959.
17 *Sad News at the Death of Sir John Crofton*. TB Alert. Available fromhttp://www/tbalert.org.news_press/News2010.php.
18 Holme, C. 'The Million Dollar Microbe', the *Glasgow Herald*, 20 May, 1989.
19 *Kenneth Murray. First Genetically Engineered Vaccine – Hepatitis B*. Available from http://www.scienceheroes.com/index.php?option=com_content&view=article&id=244&Itemid=220.
20 Will, RG *et al*. 'A New Variant of Creutzfeld-Jakob Disease in the UK', *The Lancet* 347, 1996.
21 Peden, AH *et al*. 'Preclinical vCJD After Blood Transfusion in a PRNP codon 129 Heterozygous Patient', *The Lancet* 364, 2004.
22 Wilmut I *et al*. 'Viable Offspring Derived from Fetal and Adult Mammalian Cells', *Nature*, 385, 1997.

Picture Credits

Portrait of Sophia Jex-Blake. DC.3.103. (Lothian Health Services Archive, Edinburgh University Library)

Bruntsfield Hospital. LHSA Slide Collection (LHSA/EUL/ Slide 83/12). (Lothian Health Services Archive, Edinburgh University Library)

Elsie Englis. LHSA Elsie Inglis Memorial Maternity Hospital Collection (LHSA/EUL/LHB8A/9/1). (Lothian Health Services Archive, Edinburgh University Library)

CHAPTER 5

Portrait of James Hutton. TW.1.H.66. (Edinburgh University Library, Special Collections Department)

Hutton's section of Salisbury Crags. (Photograph by George Clerk)

Geological drawing of Hutton's Section by John Clerk of Eldin. (Reproduced courtesy George Clerk)

Caricature of Joseph Black by John Kay. (The National Museum of Scotland)

Charles Darwin's matriculation class ticket for his Anatomy, Physiology and Pathology Class. EUA CA6. (Edinburgh University Library, Special Collections Department)

Old Medical School in Teviot Place (quadrangle of the University New Buildings). EUA CA1/2. (Edinburgh University Library, Special Collections Department)

Portrait of Joseph Bell. (The Royal College of Surgeons of Edinburgh)

CHAPTER 6

Watercolour of a wounded soldier at Waterloo by Charles Bell. (The Wellcome Trust)

'Section of the Brain' by Charles Bell. (The Wellcome Trust)

Portrait of John Hughes Bennett. Image held within LHSA Negative Collection (LHSA/EUL/RMS Negative Sheet 3). (The Royal Medical Society)

CHAPTER 7

Elsie Stephenson LHSA Elsie Stephenson Collection (LHSA/EUL/GD6 Photo Box 2). (Lothian Health Services Archive, Edinburgh University Library)

Students from the Polish Medical School, 1945. (The Polish School of Medicine Memorial Fund)

A medical diploma from the Polish School of Medicine. (Dr Hania Sokolowska)

Ian Wilmut and Dolly, the cloned sheep. (The Roslin Institute, University of Edinburgh)

Queen's Medical Research Institute. (The University of Edinburgh)

Index

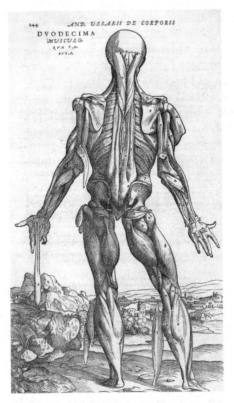

Founded in 1580, the Library has vast collections of international importance, including major resources for the history of Medicine. The 35 kilometres of Special Collections material include some significant collections of medical books and prints. There are a number of medieval manuscripts and incunabula dealing with medical issues, some beautifully illustrated. In 1763, the Royal College of Surgeons of Edinburgh gave the Library some 560 books from their historic collection. There is also a deposit of 59 very rare early medical books from the Royal Medical Society of Edinburgh. There are thousands of medical theses from the 18th century to the present day, including a special collection of some 2,000 theses presented to the great Dr Andrew Duncan (1744–1828) by grateful students. Sir John William Thomson-Walker (1871–1937), surgeon and print-collector, bequeathed some 2,500 engraved portraits of medical men. Modern medicine is also represented in the collection of 400 books from the library of pioneering psychiatrist Ronald Fairbairn (1889–1964). Veterinary Medicine is a particular strength, including a historic book collection of some 900 volumes, particularly relating to farriery.

The manuscript collections include 17th and 18th century medical treatises, notebooks and receipts, in Gaelic as well as English. There are also papers and correspondence relating to Archibald Pitcairne and Sir Robert Sibbald, two of Edinburgh's 17th century professors of medicine. From their successors in the following century the Library has lecture notes, casebooks and other material from people including Alexander Monro (primus and secundus), Charles Alston, John and James Gregory, William Cullen and Andrew Duncan (Senior). There is similar 19th century material concerning Andrew Duncan (Junior), Sir Robert Christison, Sir George Ballingall, Sir James Simpson, Thomas Laycock, John Hutton Balfour, Sir William Turner, Sir Thomas Grainger Stewart, Sir Henry Littlejohn, Lord Lister and William Rutherford. In the modern period, significant papers exist for Harvey Duncan Littlejohn, Sir Sydney Smith, Daniel John Cunningham and Norman Dott. Edinburgh medical alumni are represented in the papers of Sir James Mackenzie and the Col. John Cunningham collection on early 20th century tropical medicine.

The University Archives holds extensive collections from the various medical/scientific departments of the University. Papers of various related institutions include those from the Royal Public Dispensary, the Edinburgh Women's Medical Society, the Hunterian Medical Society, the Edinburgh Phrenological Society and the Roslin Institute.

The Lothian Health Services Archive contains much valuable material for the history of medicine in Scotland, especially the records of the Royal Infirmary of Edinburgh and the NHS in the Lothians since its creation.

There is also significant material in the University's Museum Collections, including specimens and apparatus.

The Centre for Research Collections, based on the refurbished 5th and 6th floors of the Main Library, is the main space for anyone working on these historic collections. There are extensive facilities for consultation of original material, for teaching seminars and for research and discovery. Specialist staff are available to help people locate and interpret material. These collections are accessible to anyone who needs to use them.

The Fatal Sleep

Peter Kennedy
ISBN 1 906817 48 0 PBK £9.99

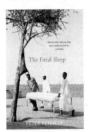

The bite of the tsetse fly – a burning sting into the skin – causes a descent into violent fever and aching pains. Severe bouts of insomnia are followed by mental deterioration, disruption of the nervous system, coma and ultimately death.

Sleeping sickness, also known as human African trypanosomiasism, is one of Africa's major killers. It puts 60 million people at risk of infection, occurs in 36 countries in sub-Saharan Africa, and claims the lives of many thousands of people every year.

Transmitted by the tsetse fly, trypanoso-miasis affects both humans and cattle. The animal form of the disease severely limits livestock production and farming, and in people the toxic effects of the treatment can be as painful and danger-ous as the disease itself.

Existing in the shadow of malaria and AIDS, it is an overlooked disease, largely ignored by pharmaceutical companies and neglected by the western world.

This is a remarkable book. It is filled in equal measure with passion for science and compassion for the people afflicted with this cruel disease.
SIR ROGER BANNISTER

The Evolution of Evolution: Darwin, Enlightenment and Scotland

Walter Stephen
ISBN 1 906817 23 5 PBK £12.99

What led Darwin to form his theory of evolution? To what extent did the Enlightenment influence Darwin's work? How did Scots help Darwin to publish the most successful and controversial book of his time?

In 1825, at the age of 16, Darwin began to study medicine at the University of Edinburgh, the seat of the Enlightenment. The Enlightenment had created a thirst for science, and in his two years at Edinburgh, Darwin became involved with the people and ideas that were to shape the world's understanding of the natural sciences. These people and theories had immense importance on the evolution of Darwin's concept of natural selection.

The Evolution of Evolution is a well researched and thoughtfully written book that recognises the importance of Scotland in the formation of evolutionary thinking and the role of Scots in both mentoring and influencing Charles Darwin throughout his life.
SCOTTISH REVIEW OF BOOKS

Luath Press Limited

committed to publishing well written books worth reading

LUATH PRESS takes its name from Robert Burns, whose little collie Luath (*Gael.*, swift or nimble) tripped up Jean Armour at a wedding and gave him the chance to speak to the woman who was to be his wife and the abiding love of his life. Burns called one of the 'Twa Dogs' Luath after Cuchullin's hunting dog in Ossian's *Fingal*. Luath Press was established in 1981 in the heart of Burns country, and is now based a few steps up the road from Burns' first lodgings on Edinburgh's Royal Mile. Luath offers you distinctive writing with a hint of unexpected pleasures.

Most bookshops in the UK, the US, Canada, Australia, New Zealand and parts of Europe, either carry our books in stock or can order them for you. To order direct from us, please send a £sterling cheque, postal order, international money order or your credit card details (number, address of cardholder and expiry date) to us at the address below. Please add post and packing as follows: UK – £1.00 per delivery address; overseas surface mail – £2.50 per delivery address; overseas airmail – £3.50 for the first book to each delivery address, plus £1.00 for each additional book by airmail to the same address. If your order is a gift, we will happily enclose your card or message at no extra charge.

Luath Press Limited

543/2 Castlehill
The Royal Mile
Edinburgh EH1 2ND
Scotland
Telephone: +44 (0)131 225 4326 (24 hours)
Fax: +44 (0)131 225 4324
email: sales@luath. co.uk
Website: www. luath.co.uk